RECIPES FOR HEALTH

Diabetes

RECIPES FOR HEALTH

Diabetes

*Low fat, low sugar, carbohydrate-counted recipes
for the management of diabetes*

AZMINA GOVINDJI AND JILL MYERS

Thorsons

Thorsons
An Imprint of HarperCollins*Publishers*
77–85 Fulham Palace Road,
Hammersmith, London W6 8JB

The website is: www.thorsonselement.com

First published as *The Essential Diabetic Cookbook* by Thorsons 1992
This edition 2000

15 17 19 21 20 18 16 14

A catalogue record for this book is
available from the British Library

ISBN-13   978-0-00-710318-8
ISBN-10   0-00-710318-2

Printed and bound in Great Britain by
Martins the Printers Ltd, Berwick upon Tweed

contents

Acknowledgements   vii
Foreword   ix

Chapter 1   What's so Special About This Book?   1
Chapter 2   Introducing Diabetes   3
Chapter 3   About the Recipes   31
Chapter 4   Soups and Starters   37
Chapter 5   Meat and Poultry   50
Chapter 6   Fish   72
Chapter 7   Vegetarian Dishes   96
Chapter 8   Salads and Side Dishes   127
Chapter 9   Puddings and Desserts   159
Chapter 10   Home Baking   181
Chapter 11   Festive Occasions   200
Chapter 12   Ideas for Children   216

Useful Addresses   229
Further Reading   233
The British Diabetic Association   234
Index   237

acknowledgements

The authors would like to thank the following people for their patience and invaluable help: Georgina West for typing the recipes; Sue Brenchley, Stella Bowling, Jane Bebell, Sue Bosanko and Judith North for their valuable comments; Elaine Messenger for putting a great deal of time and effort into evaluating the recipes; and Anise Kanji, Hanif Ladha and Joanne Winter for typing the text.

And thanks to our husbands, Shamil and Kieron, for being so tolerant!

foreword

Food is one of life's great pleasures. Having diabetes does not and need not change that. People with diabetes should know that they can enjoy any food they want. They must bear in mind just two constraints – quantity and timing.

Diabetes is having too little insulin action and, therefore, too much sugar. Food and insulin are closely linked. When the person without diabetes eats a meal, the pancreas gland automatically delivers into the bloodstream just enough insulin to process the foodstuffs for the body. People with diabetes can no longer do this. They need an 'insulin assist'. Some may be able to boost their own diminished insulin supply with a tablet, while others produce so little that they have to inject it from a syringe.

For people injecting insulin, the dose and meal need to be in balance to control and prevent wide swings – upwards or downwards – of the amount of glucose in the blood. Often, the insulin is injected just before the meal so that the two meet together. With tablets the link is not quite so close, but meal timing is important to prevent the blood glucose falling to very low levels (hypoglycaemia). For overweight people, the dietitian will advise a reducing diet – all the foods but less of them.

All this must sound complicated, even menacing to the newly diagnosed diabetic – not exactly a prescription for carefree mealtime enjoyment. However, once the initial shock has passed, a few simple facts absorbed and confidence restored, normal food and interesting meals are emphatically back on the agenda. That's when *Recipes for Health: Diabetes* comes into play. It is full of delicious dishes, aromatic advice, mouthwatering morsels. At the same time, it is a painless guide to healthy and hearty eating for the whole family.

The two authors of the book, Azmina Govindji and Jill Myers, are both very experienced in their fields. Azmina Govindji, Chief Dietitian of the British Diabetic Association, has been actively involved in the development of guidelines for diet in diabetes since 1987. As Assistant Head of the Diet Information Service, she maintains close links with government bodies, academic institutions, health professionals, food manufacturers and the media. Azmina offers advice on all matters relating to food and diabetes.

Jill Myers, formerly Home Economist to the British Diabetic Association, has considerable experience in recipe development and cookery demonstrations. While at the Association she was responsible for the production of a range of tried and tested recipes for people with diabetes and for catering establishments. She was the primary source of advice on recipe modification. Jill Myers is now working for a major food retailer as a home economist developing quality own label foods.

Whether you cook it or just eat it, with the help of this book you can look forward to pleasurable culinary ventures and enjoyable mealtimes. So, read on and *bon appetit!*

Professor Harry Keen, MD, FRCP
Chairman, Executive Council,
British Diabetic Association,
Professor Emeritus, United Medical
and Dental School, Guy's Hospital Campus

1 what's so special about this book?

You may never need another cookbook. Why not? Because this book tells you all you need to know about food now that you have diabetes. It is not just another cookery publication. This book

- is the most up-to-date cookery book for people with diabetes, incorporating all the latest dietary policies from the British Diabetic Association
- contains a wide variety of high-fibre, low-fat, low-sugar recipes that are in line with the general principles of healthy eating. This means it provides attractive recipes and essential information not only for people with diabetes, but also for anyone wishing to lose weight or to eat more healthily
- has something for everyone – the elderly who need to prepare quick, easy, and possibly cheap meals; students living on limited budgets; parents who want to provide nutritious food for the family; the keen cook who invites guests with diabetes to dinner; vegetarians and vegans; the weight watcher; and, of course, the person with diabetes

■ is a comprehensive guide to diabetes and its dietary treatment.

Sections include information on choosing the right mix of foods, healthy eating for the whole family, watching your weight, eating out, what to do in an emergency and lots more. Then there are over 200 recipes to help you put it all into practice. From soups and starters to tasty meat, fish and vegetarian dishes, this book is a must for anyone who wants to cook everyday food in an appetizing way. And who said people with diabetes shouldn't eat puddings? The mouthwatering pudding and dessert recipes will certainly prove that you need not compromise on taste just because you have diabetes!

2 introducing diabetes

What is Diabetes?

Diabetes mellitus (commonly known as diabetes) affects about two per cent of the UK population, and over 30 million people worldwide. In people with this condition, the amount of glucose in the blood is too high because the body is unable to use it properly. Glucose comes from the digestion of starchy foods such as bread or potatoes, from sugar and other sweet foods, and from the liver which makes it and passes it into the bloodstream. Insulin, a hormone produced by the pancreas, helps the glucose to enter the cells where it is used as fuel by the body.

The main symptoms of untreated diabetes are increased thirst, passing large amounts of urine, extreme tiredness, blurred vision, weight loss and itching of the genitals.

Insulin dependent diabetes (also known as Type 1 diabetes) occurs when there is a severe lack of insulin in the body because most or all of the cells which produce it have been destroyed. This type of diabetes usually appears before the age of 40. It is treated by insulin injections and diet.

Non-insulin dependent diabetes (also known as Type 2 diabetes) occurs when the body can still produce some insulin, though not enough for its needs, or when the insulin that the body does produce is not used properly by the body. This type of diabetes usually appears in people over the age of 40 and often in those who are overweight. It is treated by diet alone or by diet and tablets or, occasionally, by diet and insulin injections.

The two main aims of treatment are to eliminate the symptoms and to prevent long-term complications, such as eye, nerve, kidney and foot problems.

Diet is the foundation for the management of diabetes and the control of symptoms, and following a sensible food plan will help to keep your blood sugar close to the normal range. This in turn helps to reduce the risk of developing long-term complications. The diet for diabetes is not a special one in any way: it is a healthy eating pattern which is recommended for everyone, with or without diabetes, and one that the whole family can enjoy.

You will be able to adapt your usual meals to make them more healthy. Foods that you thought you would have to give up – such as cakes and desserts – do not need to be cut out completely. They can be eaten occasionally, as part of an overall healthy diet. Eating a variety of healthy foods can give you a sense of well-being and vitality.

The information in this book covers the basic guidelines for diabetes. For further information, contact your local Diabetic Association (see Useful Addresses, on page 229).

Don't worry if all you've heard about eating well is that carrots help you see better in the dark and spinach gives you iron – just read on.

If you have diabetes, remember to:

- continue with your treatment even if symptoms have disappeared
- attend the clinic for regular check-ups.

Your Feelings

Being told that you have a condition which will last for the rest of your life is bound to have an effect on how you organize the practical aspects of daily living and also on your feelings. It is natural for you, your family and your friends to feel sad about the loss of spontaneity that diabetes can sometimes cause. Perhaps you feel angry, asking yourself, 'Why me?' and maybe you are worried about the future.

At times like this, talking to other people who also live with diabetes can be a great help. They can share their experiences with you and give you support. The team at your diabetes clinic may be able to put you in contact with other people with diabetes. Also, your local Diabetic Association will know people who you can contact and may also arrange local support groups.

There are people with diabetes in all walks of life – from professional sports people to politicians. Some of them will work in occupations or follow interests *you* want to pursue. Although you will have to think ahead a little more than you did before, don't feel that having diabetes prevents you from having a full life.

Healthy Eating

Why is it so important to eat healthily? Research studies worldwide suggest that watching what you eat is not only essential to the management of diabetes, but that it can also help prevent heart disease, constipation, bowel problems, obesity and tooth decay. Following a good diet also makes you feel good!

There is no such thing as a bad food; there is only a bad diet. All foods can have some nutritional benefit, but it is the mix of foods and the amounts you eat that make what you eat healthy or unhealthy.

In diabetes, the nutrient value of a food is not the only consideration. The way a particular food is digested and its effect on blood sugar can influence the general control of diabetes. For example, mashed potatoes can make blood sugar rise quicker than the same amount of boiled potatoes, simply because vegetables that are left whole take longer to digest.

The following general guidelines on healthy eating will also help you to choose the right types of food. You don't need to do everything at once; start by choosing those ideas you find the easiest and gradually try to bring in the others.

- Eat regular meals and try to eat similar amounts of starchy foods from day to day.
- Try to eat more high-fibre foods. The fibre in beans, peas, lentils, vegetables, fruit and oats is particularly good.

- Cut down on fried and fatty foods such as butter, margarine, fatty meat and cheese.
- Reduce your sugar intake by swapping high-sugar foods for low-sugar foods.
- Try to get to the weight that is right for you and stay there.
- Be careful not to use too much salt.

The following suggestions will help you to put all this into practice, while the recipes in this book will enable you to prepare your favourite foods in a healthier way.

1 *Eat regular meals and try to eat similar amounts of starchy foods from day to day.* If you take insulin or tablets for your diabetes, keeping fairly closely to regular mealtimes can help to avoid hypoglycaemia (low blood sugar). Even if you do not take medication, you will find that your diabetes is easier to control if you have three or so small, regular meals a day rather than one or two large meals.

Make starchy foods (such as bread, potatoes, cereals, rice and pasta) the main part of your meal and try to eat roughly the same amounts from day to day.

2 *Try to eat more high-fibre foods.* Fibre is the part of food you don't digest. Fibre-rich foods are important for the prevention and treatment of constipation. And as they are filling and generally low in calories, they are useful if you are trying to lose weight. Fibre is found in foods such as wholemeal and wholegrain bread, jacket potatoes, wholegrain cereals, fruits and vegetables.

In diabetes, foods high in a particular type of fibre – soluble fibre – can improve blood glucose (sugar) control. Research has shown that the soluble fibre found in oats, beans and lentils can slow down the rise in blood glucose levels after a meal, so it makes sense for people with diabetes to eat these foods frequently. Soluble fibre can also reduce abnormally high blood cholesterol. Some of the recipes that follow, such as the Chickpea Moussaka (see page 105), demonstrate how you can use such foods to cook a substantial and appetizing meal.

Current nutritional thinking recommends that everyone include more fibre in their diet.

When you increase your intake of fibre, do so gradually: a new style of eating should never be adopted in haste. Drink more fluids, too, in the form of water or low-calorie drinks because your body needs plenty of fluid to digest fibrous foods. Try to drink at least six to eight cups a day.

Ways of Eating More Fibre

- Choose wholemeal, wholegrain or granary bread, vegetables with a skin (such as jacket potatoes, sweetcorn, peas), beans, lentils, brown rice and high-fibre breakfast cereals (such as porridge, muesli, bran-based cereals) in preference to more refined low-fibre foods.
- Substitute fruit juice with fresh fruit (a glass of apple juice has around 100 kcalories and no fibre whereas an apple provides only about 40 kcalories and has 2 grams of fibre).
- Choose foods as close to their natural state as possible. A food that is refined or processed generally contains less fibre. For example, white flour is lower in fibre than wholemeal flour, which has been made from the whole of the wheat grain.
- Keep high-fibre foods as whole as possible, having boiled or baked potatoes rather than mashed, and make a whole bean casserole (such as the Mixed Bean Hot Pot on page 107) instead of a puréed lentil soup. Such foods are digested more slowly and this helps to keep blood sugar levels steady.
- Try to use more beans, peas and lentils. They are cheaper than meat and are a good source of protein and fibre. Tinned baked beans are a quick way of getting more fibre and you don't even need to buy the sugar-free variety – the ordinary ones contain an insignificant amount of sugar.

Take 5!

Nutrition experts all over the world are now promoting the 'Take 5' message: take 5 portions of fruit and vegetables a day. This recommendation is based on studies which have shown that a high intake of fruit and vegetables may be associated with lower rates of heart disease and cancer. As well as soluble fibre, fruits and vegetables contain protective antioxidant vitamins – vitamins C, E and beta carotene.

Both the British Diabetic Association (BDA) and the World Health Organisation (WHO) recommend a daily intake of at least 400 grams (1 pound) of fruit and vegetables. This does not include potatoes and can be achieved by eating five portions of fruit and vegetables a day.

Choose fruit more often as an in-between meal snack and eat plenty of vegetables.

3 *Cut down on fried and fatty foods.*
A high fat intake has been shown to increase your chances of becoming obese (very overweight) or of developing heart disease. It therefore makes sense to cut down on the amount of fatty foods you eat regardless of whether or not you have diabetes. There are three main types of fat:

- saturated fats, such as dairy products, animal fats
- monounsaturated fats, such as olive oil, rapeseed oil, peanut oil
- polyunsaturated fats, such as corn oil, sunflower oil, fish oil.

Cholesterol

Cholesterol is a fatty substance that forms an essential part of the body's cells, but, equally, too much cholesterol in the body can cause problems. If the level of cholesterol in your blood is too high, you increase your chances of developing heart disease. Cholesterol can build up in the arteries (the large blood vessels) in the heart. This accumulation of cholesterol can eventually cause the arteries to become completely blocked, leading to a heart attack.

Some foods are high in cholesterol, but cutting down on these alone does not make a significant difference to blood cholesterol levels. It is more important that you cut down on the amount of *saturated* fat that you eat, as eating too much saturated fat increases your blood cholesterol level. This is particularly important for people with diabetes, as they are more prone to heart problems.

The unsaturated fats do not raise blood cholesterol in the same way that saturated fats do. Evidence now suggests that monounsaturated fats can also help keep blood cholesterol levels low. A lot of monounsaturated fat in the form of olive oil is eaten in the traditional diets of most Mediterranean countries and the rate of heart disease in these countries is low, so it would seem that the diet may be one of the factors responsible for this. Studies in other countries have also shown that healthy diets low in saturated fat and high in monounsaturated fat may reduce the risk of developing heart disease. There seems, therefore, to be an advantage in substituting foods that are high in saturated fat with polyunsaturated and monounsaturated alternatives, as well as reducing your total fat intake.

Remember that *all* fats and oils are high in calories, so use only small quantities and choose monounsaturated or polyunsaturated types whenever possible.

Fish Oils

Rates of heart disease are also low in countries where fish is eaten in large quantities. It is thought that this is because of a particular type of fat contained in fish oils. It has not yet been absolutely proved, but you certainly have nothing to lose by eating more fish. Oily fish such as mackerel, herring, salmon and trout are an excellent source of protein and of vitamins A, D and E. Try to replace some of your meat intake with fish (especially oily fish) to improve the overall quality of your diet while helping you to cut down on your total fat intake. How about making Smoked Mackerel Pâté (see page 45)?

Fats and Figures

Remember that fat is a very concentrated source of calories, so eating less fat can help you lose weight. (Calories are units used to measure the energy values of foods – see Counting Calories on page 13 for more information.) One boiled egg is approximately 70 kcalories. Have it fried and the calories almost double. A tablespoon of oil is approximately 100 kcalories – this is about the same number of calories as half a pint of beer. Think about this when you see an oily dressing on a salad!

Low-fat foods can play an important role in reducing the total amount of fat in your diet. Whether you are watching your weight, need to eat less for a specific medical condition or are simply trying to avoid a heart attack, low-fat foods can make life much easier. How-ever, be careful not to rely too heavily on some of them (such as low-fat sausages, low-fat cream cheese, low-fat crisps) because they still provide a lot of calories. Furthermore, low-fat spreads are not fat-free, so don't use twice as much! All the recipes in this book encourage low-fat cooking methods.

How to Eat Less Fat

- Try to avoid frying foods – grill, bake, boil, poach or steam instead.
- Butter and all margarines contain about the same amount of fat. Choose a reduced or low-fat monounsaturated or polyunsaturated spread. Ordinary low-fat spreads are also a good substitute for butter.
- Use lower fat versions of dairy products, for example, semi-skimmed or skimmed milk, half-fat cheddar, cottage cheese, low-fat yogurt, fromage frais.
- Cut down on fat-containing snack foods such as crisps, cakes, chocolates and biscuits.
- Buy lean meat or trim the fat off fatty meat. Poultry can be low in fat if the skin is removed. Eat fish more often. Oily fish is high in polyunsaturated fat, but, remember not to fry it!
- Watch out for processed foods that are high in fat, such as pies and other meat products – read the label.
- If you need to use oil in cooking, use as little as possible. Choose one that is high in monounsaturated fat (such as olive oil, rapeseed oil, peanut oil) or polyunsaturated fat (such as corn oil, sunflower oil, safflower oil, soya oil). Experiment with using olive oil by trying the Courgette and Sweetcorn Gratin (see page 112) or Red Lentil Lasagne (see page 100) recipes.

4. *Reduce your sugar intake by swapping high sugar foods for low sugar foods.*

It is often thought that sugar is needed for energy. However, energy is also derived from starch, protein and fat – in fact, every type of food we eat provides us with energy. All we get from sugar is calories. Sugar contains no useful nutrients nor has it any special energy-giving properties over other foods. In people with diabetes, sugary foods can cause blood glucose to rise rapidly, which is undesirable. Sugary foods can also lead to tooth decay, particularly if they are eaten between meals. Also, as sugar-containing foods are often high in fat and low in fibre, eating too many chocolates, desserts and cakes can make you put on weight.

Much of the sugar we eat is added by food manufacturers. Some packaged foods may be high in sugar even when they appear to be healthy, such as cakes and biscuits bought from health food shops. The ingredients list may not even specify sugar – but watch out for words like maltose, dextrose, honey, treacle, golden syrup, fructose, and corn syrup on the label. All of these are types of sugar and are not significantly better for you than ordinary standard sugar. Remember, too, that sucrose is simply the chemical term for ordinary standard white table sugar.

Get into the habit of reading labels and choosing foods that are low in *all* forms of sugar. If an item is low down on the ingredients list, there is less of that ingredient in the food than the ingredients given before it.

Sugar can cause tooth decay and eating too many sugary foods can make you put on weight, so eat less sugar.

Sugar and Diabetes – Putting it into Context

People with diabetes are advised to avoid drinks containing sugar. Because the sugar in these drinks is in liquid form, it can enter the blood quite quickly. This causes blood sugar to rise rapidly. With diabetes, you want to avoid this.

However, if sugar is taken mixed in with food (such as an ice-cream after a meal), then blood sugar rises more slowly. So, if you wish to eat a small amount of sweet food, such as a piece of cake or a dessert, then try to have it after a meal.

Cutting Down on Sugar

- Try not to add sugar to drinks or cereals. There is a range of artificial sweeteners that make excellent substitutes (see Artificial Sweeteners, below).
- Choose unsweetened fruit juice, and diet or low-calorie drinks rather than sweetened soft drinks. One 330ml can of a sweetened fizzy drink can contain 7 teaspoons of sugar!
- Buy reduced-sugar jams, pure fruit spreads and fruit tinned in natural juice instead of their sweetened alternatives.
- Save cakes, sweets and chocolates for special occasions only.
- Look at labels and try to avoid manufactured foods that contain a lot of sugar.

Artificial Sweeteners – not Sugar, but Sweet

Artificial sweeteners have made an enormous range of foods readily available for all those who want to avoid large quantities of sugar – slimmers, the health conscious and people with diabetes. They impart an intense level of sweetness and are virtually calorie-free. Available as tablets, liquids or in granulated form, they can be used to replace sugar in drinks, cereals and puddings. They are also found in many reduced-calorie foods such as diet yogurts, low-calorie squash and diet soft drinks.

All these artificial substitutes for sugar are food additives and so are required by law to undergo rigorous tests for safety before being approved for use. Examples of those commonly used are aspartame, saccharin, and acesulfame potassium (acesulfame K). All of these are widely available under various brand names. Neohesperidine (NHDC) is the newest permitted sweetener in this country. Cyclamate is widely sold in Europe and may receive approval for sale in the UK.

Personal preferences vary, so it is a good idea to shop around until you find one that suits your palate and your pocket best – the prices also vary! If you tend to use a lot of sweeteners in drinks, cereals, puddings and processed foods, make sure you vary the type of sweetener you choose so as to reduce any chance of over-consumption of one food additive.

Unlike sugar, artificial sweeteners do not cause tooth decay and are virtually calorie-free.

5 *Try to get to the weight that is right for you and stay there.*
  If you are underweight, you may not be getting all the nutrients you need. If you are overweight, your diabetes will be harder to control.

Counting Calories

What Are Calories?

The term 'calories' or 'kcalories' (kilocalories) is used to describe the amount of energy provided by the food you eat. All food provides calories but some foods are more concentrated in calories than others. For example, a 100g/4oz apple will provide you with around 50 kcalories, whereas a 100g/4oz piece of Cheddar cheese would provide 400 kcalories. This is because every food contains a different proportion of fat, carbohydrate and protein. Weight for weight, fat contains twice as many calories as either carbohydrate or protein. Therefore, those foods that have a higher percentage of fat are likely to be highest in calories.

On food labels, the calorific value of a food is usually written as kcal/100g. For example, if a label states 350 kcals/100g then this means that a 100g/4oz portion of the food would provide 350 kcalories. You may also see the term kilojoule (kj) used on labels. One kcalorie is equal to 4.2kj.

If the number of calories you take in from the food you eat is the *same* as the number you use up in your daily activities, your weight should be more or less stable. However, if you take in *more* calories from food than you use up, you are likely to gain weight. On the other hand, if you eat *less* than normal but maintain your usual level of activity, you may lose weight.

Why Count Calories?

Being overweight can increase your chances of developing diabetes, heart disease and high blood pressure. If you have diabetes and are overweight, weight reduction can improve the control of your diabetes and may even mean that you can reduce the dosage of your medication.

Motivation

Why is it that at some time in their lives most people have tried some sort of slimming diet, that the bookshops are oozing with novel ideas on how to shed those extra pounds and yet obesity is *still* a major problem in most Western countries?

From the restricted grapefruit diet (not to be encouraged) to the more sensible high-fibre, low-fat type of diet, you are presented with hundreds of ways to cut down on calories. Often one of these will help you lose weight but, more often than not, the weight starts to creep back on again. There are, no doubt, many reasons for this, but one of the most important is motivation – or lack of it. If you can maintain your motivation, then you are more likely to make a concerted effort to persevere. How, though, can you keep yourself motivated? It is unlikely that you will keep to a diet if it makes unreasonable demands on your normal lifestyle. Only if your new way of eating fits in with your social habits, your time constraints, your budget and your food preferences will you have a strong chance of keeping your weight down for a significant length of time.

Support

Reputable commercial slimming clubs can provide invaluable personal support as you try to lose weight. Most people who are trying to lose weight need guidance on more than just what to put on their plates at mealtimes. Psychological and emotional support can make changing your eating behaviour much easier and often these clubs can provide a degree of one-to-one counselling.

In some cases, your doctor may refer you to the state registered dietitian at the local hospital or clinic. A qualified dietitian will take your medical history, age, sex and lifestyle into account and will then be able to help you with a personal food plan. This can vary from person to person. The dietitian can, in addition, offer guidance and support as necessary.

If you follow the general guidelines on healthy eating given on pages 5–7 you will be able to adopt a style of eating that will help you lose weight while still providing you with all the nutrients you need. If you choose the foods you eat sensibly and cook them in the ways suggested in this book, you will be able to reduce your calorie intake and still enjoy tasty, filling meals.

Sensible slimming suggestions

- Be realistic when deciding how much weight you want to lose – setting a goal that seems unattainable could make you feel frustrated and give up.
- Set short-term targets and reward yourself once you've reached them. For example, treat yourself to a record or a book after you've lost 7 lb (about 3kg). Don't use food as a reward, though, or you'll undo all your good work!
- Try recording *exactly* what you eat – you may be surprised to see how the nibbles and snacks mount up.
- Make changes slowly. For example, try to avoid fried foods one week and, then, in the following week, to eat high-fibre breakfast cereals as well.
- Write down your successes – this can help keep you motivated.
- Try to encourage your family to eat healthily. This way you won't need to prepare foods specifically for yourself, you will simply need to have smaller portions.
- Think of ways to help your meals appear larger. Use a smaller plate, or have a selection of vegetables.
- Try to avoid TV dinners as concentrating on TV can make you less aware of how much you're eating. Try to sit down when you are eating – it's amazing how much you can munch your way through on the move!
- Don't shop when you're hungry – you may be tempted into buying more than you need (using a shopping list is a good idea) and avoid the aisles full of sweets and biscuits and the cakes at the in-store bakery!

Are You Overweight?

It's obviously worth finding out if you *need* to lose weight before you start slimming. Use the chart on page 16 to estimate how much (if any) weight you need to lose. Remember not to make unreasonable demands on yourself. Aim to get down to a weight that is practical and possible. Don't bother to weigh yourself every day as you may find you lose one day and gain the next.

This is normal, but can be disheartening. Try to weigh yourself only once a week and at around the same time of day.

Diets that offer a weight loss of 7 lb (3kg) in a week may sound like a miracle cure, but will not help you in the long term. So be patient – it took time to gain the excess weight, so losing it effectively is going to take time, too. The ideal rate of weight loss is around 1–2 lb (½–1kg) per week, although there is often a rapid loss in the beginning (mostly of water). A steady weight loss of around 4 lb (2kg) per month is good.

As time goes on your body adapts to your new calorie intake by needing fewer calories for normal functions such as breathing. Don't be discouraged, keep at it. Keep up the motivation, maintain variety, experiment with new recipes, reward yourself (but not with food) when you have done well, exercise, eat out (sensibly) on occasions, take up a new hobby, diet with a friend or whatever else helps. Do everything within your power to get down to that target weight – it will be worth it.

Weight Chart

Take a straight line across from your height (without shoes) and a line up from your weight (without clothes). Mark where the two lines meet.

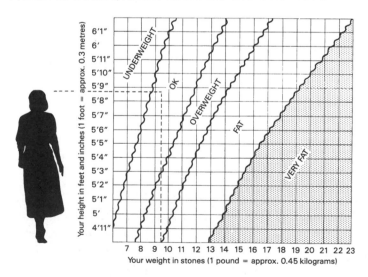

From Garrow JS (1981), *Treat Obesity Seriously*. Edinburgh: Churchill Livingstone.

Underweight Maybe you need to eat a bit more, but go for well-balanced nutritious foods and don't just fill up on fatty and sugary foods. If you are *very* underweight, see your doctor about it.

OK You're eating the right *quantity* of food but you need to be sure that you're getting a healthy *balance* in your diet.

Overweight You should try to lose weight.

Fat You need to lose weight.

Very fat You urgently need to lose weight. You would do well to see your doctor, who might refer you to a dietitian.

If you need to lose weight, aim to lose 1 or 2 lb (½–1kg) a week until you get down to the 'OK' range. Go for fibre-rich foods and cut down on fat, sugar and alcohol. You'll need to take regular exercise too.

Use the recipes in this book to help you follow the healthy eating guidelines. Each recipe has been given a calorie value to help you keep track of how much you are eating.

If you have insulin dependent diabetes, changing your diet may mean you have to inject less insulin. It is best to consult your doctor and dietitian before adopting a reduced calorie, and probably carbohydrate, diet.

What happens next? Often after getting your weight down successfully, it slowly starts to creep up again as you allow yourself more treats. Once you are satisfied with your weight, gradually include more variety, especially of the high fibre starchy foods. Start, for example, by having an extra slice of bread or an extra helping of potatoes and then slowly introduce more of the other foods you enjoy. Continue to step on the scales regularly so that you can keep your new weight in check.

Lastly, good luck – you *can* do it!

6 *Be careful not to use too much salt.*

Most experts on nutrition advise you to eat less salt. Why?

In some people, eating salt may be linked with high blood pressure. Although a small amount of salt is needed by the body, it is possible for the average person to eat up to ten times more salt than the body requires. A lot of the salt we eat is added by the manufacturers during food processing. Cutting down on processed food can therefore help you to eat less salt.

Cutting Down on Salt

■ Use less salt in cooking (experiment with other seasonings, such as herbs and spices).
■ Avoid adding salt at the table.
■ Eat fewer salty manufactured foods, such as smoked and preserved meat and fish, sausages and salted snack foods.

What about Alcohol?

Weight for weight, alcohol contains more calories than sugar, so even moderate drinking can make you gain weight. For example, one pint of beer has about the same number of calories as three chocolate biscuits. Also, as alcohol contains negligible nutrients, it is of little dietary benefit. Replacing meals with alcoholic drinks can make you lose out on important vitamins and minerals. If you have diabetes, you don't need to give up drinking alcohol altogether, but you do need to think more carefully about what you drink and when.

Alcohol in large quantities can damage your liver. The recommended maximum intake for anyone, with or without diabetes, is 3 units of alcohol for men and 2 units for women. Try to have two or three drink-free days each week. Pregnant and breastfeeding women should ideally avoid alcoholic drinks altogether.

The above all contain one unit of alcohol.

Use the guidelines below to help you keep your social drinking to safe limits.

- Do not exceed the recommended maximum intakes.
- Try low-sugar, low-alcohol drinks – they are better for your blood glucose (important if you have diabetes) and for your waistline.
- Never drink on an empty stomach; eat before you drink.
- Alternate your alcoholic drinks with alcohol-free drinks. If drinking spirits, use sugar-free mixers or soda water.
- Remember not to drink and drive.

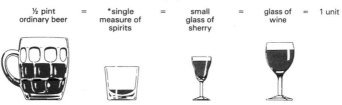

These drinks all contain roughly the same amount of alcohol.

½ pint ordinary beer = *single measure of spirits = small glass of sherry = glass of wine = 1 unit

*In Northern Ireland a single measure of spirits = 1½ units.

If you have diabetes, you should also note the following:

- you may drink up to three units of sweet wine or sherry as part of your weekly allowance, but try not to drink them all on the same occasion

- you should avoid the special low-carbohydrate beers and lagers that were originally brewed for people with diabetes – they are higher in alcohol and calories than ordinary beers

- it is important to wear some form of diabetic identification – you and others may confuse low blood sugar (hypoglycaemia) with drunkenness

- alcohol lowers blood sugar, so remember this, particularly if you are on insulin. This (hypoglycaemic) effect can last several hours

- if you count how much carbohydrate (CHO) you eat, don't include the CHO from alcoholic drinks.

About Carbohydrate

The amount of carbohydrate (CHO) or starchy foods eaten daily is an important consideration for people with diabetes. It is often felt that people with diabetes should cut down on starchy foods. This is not true. In the past, a low CHO diet was encouraged. However, it has since been shown that if around half your daily calorie intake comes from high-CHO, high-fibre foods, then your blood sugar level will improve. This is obviously better in the long term. The starchy foods recommended in the section on fibre on pages 5–7 are the best types to choose. The soluble fibre they contain has the most favourable effect on blood glucose and may also help reduce blood cholesterol levels.

Latest Developments

Many studies have been conducted in this field and you may hear rumours that this amount of CHO can make your control worse, instead of improving it. Don't worry! After an extensive review of all the research that has been published, the British Diabetic Association still recommends that a high-CHO, low-fat diet is the most appropriate for people with diabetes, *provided the diet is high in soluble fibre*, particularly in its whole, unprocessed form. The Canadian, Australian, American and European Associations also encourage a high-CHO, high-fibre, low-fat diet.

What is a 'CHO exchange'?

All meals eaten by people with diabetes must contain some CHO. To help people with diabetes control their CHO intake and still enjoy varied and interesting meals, a system of 'exchanges' has been developed. An exchange refers to a particular amount of CHO. One apple and one orange each contain approximately 10g of CHO, and can thus be 'exchanged', or swapped, for one another.

CHO 'exchange lists' are used by some insulin dependent diabetics, but they can be impractical. Many people prefer to use ordinary household measures (cups, spoons and so on) to weigh food. It may be that general advice on the quantity of the diet and the best mix of foods will eventually replace the CHO counting system. Placing so much emphasis on CHO is considered by many experts to be misleading as CHO is not the only nutrient that you need to adjust when you have diabetes. Far more important is the *whole diet*: the mix of foods that are eaten and when, how long they are cooked and whether they are puréed or eaten whole.

Exchange lists are, however, still very much in use. In Canada and America, in fact, up to nine food exchange lists may be used. The European Association for the Study of Diabetes, while currently recommending CHO exchange systems, acknowledges that better exchange lists should be developed. These lists should encourage the use of the more beneficial type of CHO, high-soluble fibre carbohydrates.

Each recipe in this book has been given a carefully calculated CHO value – this will be useful to you if your dietitian has prescribed a daily CHO allowance.

Use this book to ensure that you select the foods that are the most appropriate for good control of your diabetes and also for good health.

Diabetic Products

These specialist products have been on the market since the 1960s. At that time, the diabetic diet strictly prohibited the consumption of sugar and a low carbohydrate intake was encouraged. Because of this, special diabetic foods that were sugar-free and low in carbohydrate were considered to be a good idea.

Times change, however, and, as we learn more about nutrition, so do recommended diets. Today a high-carbohydrate, high-fibre diet is recommended and a small amount of sugar is acceptable, provided that it forms part of this diet. So treats can now include ordinary chocolates, cakes or biscuits, so long as they are eaten in small amounts within the context of a healthy diet, preferably at the end of a meal. Useful proprietary products that are not marketed especially for people with diabetes are sugar-free drinks, diet yogurts and artificial sweeteners.

So, you don't *need* to buy or eat special diabetic products. Because they also tend to be expensive and are often no lower in fat or calories than their non-diabetic equivalents, consuming them is now discouraged in many countries.

Making Meals

You now know which foods are the better ones to choose and which foods to cut down on; you will shortly learn which cooking methods to adopt and have a selection of tasty recipes, but how do you transform all this knowledge and information into practical food terms? How do you 'make meals'?

On the next page is an example of a day's food intake. Have a go at changing the foods chosen and the cooking methods so that the meals are healthier and more appropriate for people with diabetes. Compare your suggestions to the ones on pages 23–4.

A day's food

Breakfast
Cornflakes with whole
milk and sugar
White toast with butter
and jam
Coffee with milk and sugar

Lunch
2 slices white bread with
Cheddar cheese, tomato
and mayonnaise
Banana
Sugary fizzy drink, such
as Coke

Mid-afternoon snack
2 chocolate biscuits
Tea with milk and sugar

Supper
Shepherd's pie
Cabbage
Fruit crumble
Custard

Bedtime
Tea with milk and sugar

Healthier choices

_____

_____
_____

_____
_____

_____

_____
_____

_____
_____
_____
_____

_____

Healthier choices	Comments
Breakfast	
Breakfast cereal containing bran or porridge or muesli	■ more fibre ■ oats contain soluble fibre
Semi-skimmed or skimmed milk	■ less fat
Granulated artificial sweetener	■ sugar free
Wholemeal or granary toast	■ whole grains may help keep blood sugar at a safe level
Polyunsaturated or monounsaturated margarine or low-fat spread	■ less saturated fat ■ less total fat and fewer calories
Reduced-sugar jam or pure fruit spread	■ less sugar ■ fewer calories
Coffee with semi-skimmed or skimmed milk	■ less fat
Artificial sweetener	■ sugar free
Lunch	
2 slices wholemeal or granary bread	■ more fibre
Low-fat or half-fat cheddar or cottage cheese or Edam cheese	■ less fat
Tomato	
Reduced-calorie mayonnaise	■ less fat and fewer calories
Banana	
Diet fizzy drink (such as diet Coke or equivalent)	■ sugar free and fewer calories

Mid-afternoon snack
2 plain biscuits

■ less sugar, less fat and fewer calories

Tea with semi-skimmed
or skimmed milk
Artificial sweetener

■ less fat and fewer calories
■ sugar free

Supper
Lean savoury mince
Boiled or baked potatoes
in their jackets
Sweetcorn
Fruit crumble, sweetened
with artificial sweetener
and crumble topping made
from wholemeal flour,
muesli, poly- or mono-
unsaturated margarine or
low-fat spread

■ less fat
■ more fibre
■ vegetables kept whole
■ more soluble fibre

■ sugar free

■ more fibre (muesli has soluble fibre)
■ less saturated fat or less total fat

Bedtime
Tea with semi-skimmed or
skimmed milk
Artificial sweetener

■ less fat
■ sugar free

As you can see, only small changes have been made, but by choosing low-fat, high-fibre, low-sugar foods and by adopting sensible cooking methods, the health giving quality of the meals has been greatly improved. Use this guide and the practical cooking tips on pages 5–7 to help you make all your meals more healthy.

The Plate Model – The Latest Approach

You eat foods, not nutrients. It is helpful to translate all this advice into what you actually put on your plate. For this reason, many health experts, including the British Diabetic Association, have issued guidelines on how much of your plate should be filled by individual foods. Such an approach provides a visual guide to meal planning.

Always make starchy foods such as bread, potatoes, rice, pasta or cereals the main part of your meal. More than a third of your plate should be covered by this filling starchy food (see plate diagram below). Around the same amount of your plate should contain vegetables (and/or fruit). The remainder of your plate is left for the protein foods, such as meat, fish, cheese or eggs. This amounts to about a quarter of the area on your plate and will help you to cut down on fat and calories. Even if you are not concerned about your calorie intake, these proportions are considered to be ideal for general health.

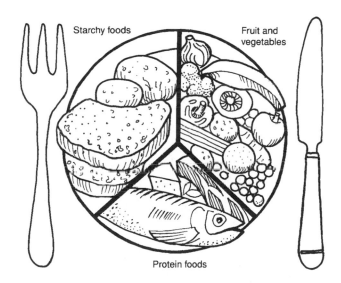

Eating Away From Home

If you have diabetes, there is no reason why you can't visit the local fast food joint, the posh restaurant in town, go to your friend's house for dinner or a holiday resort abroad.

A Quick Take-Away

As with any food or drink, it makes sense to limit the amount of 'fast food' you eat. It does have the benefit of being quick and convenient, so avoiding it altogether can be a nuisance. Simply try not to rely on such foods too often and, when you do, make the most healthy choice possible. For example, choose a smaller hamburger in a wholemeal bun, if available, and unsweetened orange juice or a diet drink. Try to resist that sugary, processed apple pie. They are often more like apple fritters than pies and can be incredibly high in fat. Remember, too, that one milkshake can have more calories than seven wine glasses of fresh orange juice!

The Chinese stir-fry is becoming an increasingly popular fast-food choice. These foods are generally healthy, particularly since a wide variety of vegetables make up an important part of the meal. Obviously the oily dishes such as deep fried seaweed, spring rolls, fried prawn balls, crispy Peking duck and fried noodles can be very high in fat, and steamed alternatives are preferable. The main meals generally contain very little carbohydrate and only the rice and noodle dishes need to be counted if you are on a daily carbohydrate allowance. Sweet and sour dishes are best kept for special occasions. They tend to be high in fat, sugar and calories.

The Greek doner kebab may look lean, but have you noticed the oil that trickles down the outside? Don't believe you have lost all of the fat in this way, there is still 'hidden' fat in the meat. Lower fat choices are grilled kebabs, especially chicken. Fill some hot pitta bread (preferably wholemeal) with kebabs and a colourful salad for a filling, nutritious and convenient meal.

The local 'chippy' unfortunately does not have many healthy foods on offer since most items are deep fried or contain pastry. Ordering a couple of rolls and less of the fatty food can be helpful.

The tempting aroma emanating from an Indian restaurant can act like a magnet when you are hungry! Choose lentil (or dahl) based dishes, tandooris and grills, naan or chapati (unbuttered) and boiled rice. Save high fat dishes like fried poppadums, butter chicken, paratha (deep fried Indian bread) and biryani or pilau rice for special occasions. Did you know that an average portion of pilau rice has more than double the calories of a portion of plain boiled rice?

Dining in Style

What about a night out at an exclusive restaurant? On a special occasion, why not enjoy yourself and eat what you like? If it is your birthday, anniversary, Christmas, whatever, do you think it will do you much harm to forget the fat and fibre for just one evening? If you want a small serving of dessert, remember that sugar has a less drastic effect on your blood sugar level when it is mixed in with lots of other ingredients and eaten at the end of a meal. (Remember if you take insulin, though, that you may need to make some adjustments – see page 28.)

If you eat out frequently, however, perhaps attending business lunches or spending three nights a week wining and dining, then you need to think more carefully about the foods you choose. Try to avoid rich, creamy sauces, fried foods and sweet, fattening desserts. Watch the amount of alcohol you have, too.

Guess Who's Coming to Dinner?

When a friend invites you to dinner, don't forget that other people's knowledge of diabetes and food may be limited. If you feel that you would like to plan ahead, it may be worth letting your host or hostess know which foods you would prefer to be served – perhaps some of the mouthwatering dishes from this book! Otherwise, simply select whatever you think best from the dining table and, remember, an occasional lapse from your diet is not detrimental.

Sun, Sand, Sea – and Food

A little thoughtful planning before setting off for a week in the sun can make an important difference to your trip. Many people nowadays prefer self-catering accommodation, which will obviously mean that you have maximum control over what you eat. However, hotels often have a reasonable choice on the menu. If you are confronted with a range of unusual foods you are not sure about, you can almost always ask for bread, pasta or rice with a simple accompaniment like an omelette or cheese until you have discovered exactly what is on offer.

Remember to take extra carbohydrate supplies with you on the journey to your holiday destination. Suitable convenience snacks include sandwiches, fruit, biscuits and crisps. Take emergency supplies of glucose tablets or sweets along as well.

Insulin and Carbohydrate when eating out

If you take insulin, adjustments may need to be made to:

- your preceding snack or meal
- your insulin dose
- the timing of your injection.

You will probably work out what sort of changes are required by trial and error, but the following tips may be useful:

- plan ahead whenever possible
- extra carbohydrate (CHO) does need extra insulin (the dose depends on how much CHO is in the food)
- extra insulin is usually taken in the form of a quick-acting insulin shortly before a meal – this is particularly helpful if the meal is served later than you had anticipated
- you could delay the timing of your insulin injection if your meal is due to be taken later than usual
- if you are eating late, you could try having a snack at your usual mealtime to prevent your blood sugar from falling too low before your main meal
- if you use a pen injector, you will have a greater degree of flexibility – you can assess the CHO value of your meal and inject accordingly
- if you are dining and dancing, remember that the energy you use up while dancing will lower your blood sugar and, consequently, you may need to inject less insulin or eat more carbohydrate
- alcohol lowers blood sugar. Normally this is not a problem, but if you take insulin, it is important to have some food before or with an alcoholic drink and, most importantly, afterwards (such as a bedtime snack). This will prevent your blood sugar level falling too low, as the effect of alcohol can last for several hours.

Emergency Measures for Low Blood Sugar

The medical term for a low blood sugar level is hypoglycaemia or a hypo. Hypos are most likely to occur in people who inject insulin, but some people on certain tablets may also experience a hypo. It can be caused by:

- missing a meal or snack
- eating less carbohydrate than usual
- engaging in strenuous activity that you have not compensated for by, for example, eating some carbohydrate
- injecting more insulin than you need
- drinking alcohol on an empty stomach.

Please don't feel that you have to look for a cause, however, as there may be no obvious reason.

Signs and symptoms of hypoglycaemia vary from one person to the next, but common ones include light-headedness, a faint feeling, sweating, shaking, hunger and confusion. You will soon learn the warning signs of a hypo and it is a good idea to let a friend or relative know what these are, too, so that they can recognize one.

What to Do if You Have a Hypo

The main aim is to raise your blood sugar level quickly. The fastest way to do this is to have some form of concentrated sugar (see the list on page 30 for examples) immediately, followed by a snack, such as a slice of bread, biscuits or milk.

Carry something from the list below with you at all times. Wearing some sort of diabetic identification is an effective way of telling people you don't know around you that you have diabetes, should you need further help in such instances. If you cannot swallow, a doctor or ambulance should be called immediately. If you know why the hypo occurred, try to make adjustments to prevent it happening again. Seek the advice of your doctor, diabetes specialist nurse or dietitian if necessary.

Illness

When you are ill, you may not feel like eating. However, even if you do not eat any food, you will find that your blood sugar level tends to go up when you are ill. Your body naturally responds to illness by making more sugar. It is obviously very important, therefore, to *continue with your diabetic treatment*. The following suggestions may also be useful:

- consult your doctor, particularly if you are vomiting
- if you are not eating, take fluids such as fruit juice, soup or a glucose drink (such as Lucozade), with 'a little and often' being a good motto – for example, half a glass every hour
- if you are eating, have small, frequent meals
- if possible, test your blood sugar or urine at least four times a day and keep a record of the results
- if you take insulin, the dose may need adjusting – for example, if your blood sugar is very high, you will need more insulin (call your doctor if you need help with this).

Suggested emergency items	Amount to take
Glucose tablets	3 tablets
Sugar or glucose powder	2 teaspoons
Sugar cubes	2 cubes
Honey, jam or syrup	2 teaspoons
Lucozade or similar glucose drink	50ml/2fl oz
Sugared fizzy drink, such as ordinary coca-cola	½ glass
Orange juice	½ glass

3 about the recipes

All the recipes in this book have been prepared in a healthy way. High-fibre, low-fat ingredients have been used and low-fat cooking methods have been chosen. Each recipe has been carefully tried and tested. The calorie and carbohydrate content of each recipe has been accurately calculated using the latest professional nutrition data.

The Ingredients Used

Fat

- wherever possible, polyunsaturated and monounsaturated oils (try to use monounsaturated oils more often)
- low-fat spread (including polyunsaturated low-fat spread)
- lean meat and poultry or low-fat dairy products.

Fibre

- lentils, beans, wholemeal pasta, brown rice, wholemeal flour, oats, dried fruit, fresh fruit and vegetables.

Sugar

- small amounts of ordinary sugar in baking
- artificial sweeteners in desserts where sugar is not required.

Weights and Measures

Quantities of ingredients have been given in both metric and imperial measurements. The metric measurements have been used for the calculations. Choose whichever system of measurement you prefer, but use either *all* metric or *all* imperial, otherwise you risk a poor result, especially with pastry, breads and cakes.

Recipe Calculations

All calculations are based on raw ingredients, unless the word 'cooked' appears in the ingredient list.

Carbohydrate (CHO) Calculations

The section about carbohydrate on page 19 explained why CHO is important in diabetes. Not all foods contain CHO. For example, many vegetables – such as lettuce, tomato, carrots and cabbage – and fruits – such as rhubarb, lemons, raspberries and gooseberries – have such small amounts of CHO that it does not make sense to count them. The same is true for flavourings such as stock and tomato purée. If a food contains less than 5g of CHO, it is considered negligible (referred to as 'neg.' in the recipes). The list below is of the vegetables that have been counted when making CHO calculations for the recipes in this book:

- baked beans
- pulses and beans, such as chickpeas, split peas, lentils
- potatoes.

It is more practical to round up or down to the nearest 10g rather than to use the exact CHO value. For example if a recipe has 23g of CHO per portion, this has been rounded down to 20g. This makes CHO counting much easier.

Calorie calculations

All foods provide calories, but in some cases the number of calories is so minute that it is not necessary to count them. In this book, seasonings, certain condiments (such as vinegar and lemon juice) and artificial sweeteners have not been calorie counted.

Although some vegetables (such as cabbage and carrots) are very low in calories, their calorie content has been included in the recipe calculations to make them as accurate as possible. However, on a day-to-day basis the calories from these vegetables need not be counted, so eat them freely.

As with CHO, the exact calorie content of the ingredients has been assessed. The total figure for the recipe has then been rounded up or down to the nearest 10 kcalories.

Adapting Your Own Recipes For Home Baking

No one is suggesting that you should throw away all your favourite recipes and cookbooks just because you are now following a healthy eating plan. Instead, modify them by reducing the amount of saturated fat and sugar they contain and increasing the amount of fibre. You may find the following guidelines useful:

- if a recipe calls for white flour, try using wholemeal flour instead or half wholemeal and half white. This gives a lighter texture than wholemeal on its own for sponge cakes and so on
- replacing butter and ordinary margarine with low-fat spread can reduce the fat and calories by half, but some of these spreads do not work well in baking, so polyunsaturated or monounsaturated margarines are a useful alternative. (Remember, however, that

these margarines have exactly the same quantity of fat and calories as ordinary butter, although they do have the advantage of being high in unsaturated fat so using a polyunsaturated or monounsaturated low-fat spread gives you the best of both worlds; look out, too, for new low-fat products designed especially for baking)

■ in most cases, you can reduce the sugar content of a traditional recipe (such as for a Victoria sandwich) by half: proportions of up to 50g/2oz of sugar to 225g/8oz of flour give satisfactory results in rock cakes, scones, fruit loaves and so on and, on average, this yields between 2 and 5g of sugar per scones, which is the same as a couple of digestive biscuits

■ remember that if you use sugar, it does add to the carbohydrate content of a recipe

■ not everyone needs to count their calories and CHO and you are certainly not expected to own food composition tables such as those that have been used in the compiling of this book, but if you are on a CHO allowance, the table below may be of help.

Ingredients	CHO (in grams)
25g/1oz flour (any kind)	20
25g/1oz sugar (any kind)	30
Polyunsaturated margarine or low-fat spread	No carbohydrate content
Eggs	No carbohydrate content
185ml/⅓ pint of milk (any kind)	10
25g/1oz dried fruit (any kind)	20
Up to 100g/4oz nuts	Negligible carbohydrate content
Up to 50g/2oz cocoa powder	Negligible carbohydrate content

Practical Cooking Tips

- Try baking cakes using less sugar than a traditional recipe demands. In some cases you can use only half the normal amount and still concoct a mouthwatering treat. How about a Victoria Sandwich (see page 183) for a high-fibre, low-sugar accompaniment to afternoon tea?
- If making custard, use skimmed milk, custard powder and an artificial sweetener.
- Make your own jelly using low-calorie squash, unsweetened fruit juice and gelatine.
- Include beans, peas and lentils in recipes that contain meat. Replacing some of the meat with beans is cheaper and very nutritious.
- Use reduced or low-fat spread, preferably monounsaturated (if available) or polyunsaturated, for baking – try the Banana and Walnut Slices on page 186). Use non-stick cookware, too.
- Remove the skin from poultry and trim the fat off meat.
- Choose refreshing fruity desserts such as the Raspberry and Kiwi Whip on page 166, rather than rich stodgy puds.
- Reduce the amount of salt you use in cooking as we eat far more salt than we need. Flavour your food with lemon juice, herbs, spices or mustard instead for healthier, tastier food.
- Eat more oily fish, such as herring and mackerel, that are high in polyunsaturated fat and are still moist after grilling.
- Grill, bake, poach, steam or boil foods rather than frying them. 25g/1oz of boiled potato provides about 20 kcalories – make this amount of potato into chips and the calories multiply three times!
- Choose oils that are high in monounsaturated fat (such as olive oil) or polyunsaturated fat (such as corn oil) and, even so, remember to use as little as possible. Also, remember that polyunsaturated oil becomes more saturated when it is reused, which makes it less desirable in your diet, but that monounsaturated oils are not altered when they are reused. So, when frying, choose a monounsaturated oil if you are planning to reuse it.

- Use low-fat dairy products in recipes, such as skimmed or semi-skimmed milk, reduced-fat cheese and low-fat yogurt. Low-fat cream cheese and low-fat yogurt make good substitutes for cream. How about making the Yogurt Gooseberry Fool on page 167?
- Beans don't necessarily need to be the dried variety, which require soaking. Canned beans are just as healthy and can be used straight away.
- Keep the skins on potatoes. This doesn't mean having potatoes baked in their jackets day in, day out – roasted, scalloped, sautéd or boiled potatoes can all be cooked with their skins on and you benefit from the extra fibre.
- Brown rice contains more fibre than white. Try it sometime. (Remember, though, that you need more water for brown rice and it takes longer to cook.)
- Use half wholemeal and half white flour for baking – you don't need to use wholemeal on its own, which can be quite dry in some baked goods. Simply choose what you and your family find tastes good.

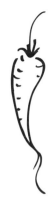

4 soups and starters

An enticing starter often paves the way for good things to come. Starters should complement the main course. It's best to serve small portions and to present them attractively with eye-catching garnishes.

Cold starters can be prepared in advance, enabling you to deal with other parts of the meal or to take part in the socializing! Serve pâtés or dips with raw, fresh vegetables such as carrots, celery and cauliflower florets to help add fibre and colour.

Delicious, home-made soups are always welcoming on a cold winter's day. They are extremely nourishing and can be transformed into a light main meal if served with wholegrain granary rolls or bread. The use of vegetables and pulses in the soups helps to increase the fibre and adds texture.

Taramasalata

▶ CHO 80g ▶ CALORIES 940   *serves 8–10*

8 small slices wholemeal bread
175g/6oz/1 cup fresh smoked cod roe, skinned
juice of 1–2 lemons
1 slice onion
1 clove garlic, crushed
50ml/2fl oz/¼ cup oil
olives, to garnish

1   Soak the bread in water for 10 minutes. Squeeze it gently then put it in a food processor or blender.
2   Add the roe, lemon juice, onion and garlic. Blend for 2 minutes until well mixed.
3   Slowly add the oil while the blender is running. Blend for 1–2 minutes.
4   Serve with brown pitta bread and vegetable crudités.

▶ *Notes to Cooks If a milder taste is preferred, add a little more bread and oil. If it is too stiff, add 1–2 teaspoons water. The consistency should be neither runny nor too stiff, but rather, a spreadable consistency.*

Vegetable crudités is the French name for a dish of raw vegetables, including carrots, celery, cauliflower, peppers, radishes etc., usually cut into sticks and served with one or more dips or sauces as an appetizer or cocktail snack.

Minestrone Soup

▶ CHO 50g ▶ CALORIES 790 *serves 6–8*

1 x 15ml sp/1 tbs olive oil
75g/3oz/3 slices rindless streaky bacon, chopped
1 onion, chopped
1 clove garlic, crushed
3 stalks celery, chopped
2 small carrots, finely chopped
1 courgette, chopped
25g/1oz/$^{1}/_{4}$ cup small dried pasta shells, bows or similar
salt and freshly ground black pepper
1 x 5ml sp/1 tsp dried oregano or basil
1 x 15ml sp/1 tbs tomato purée
1.1ltr/2 pints /5 cups chicken stock
225g/1 x 8oz can/1$^{1}/_{4}$ cups red kidney beans, drained and refreshed
under cold running water
a little grated Parmesan cheese

1   Heat the oil in a large saucepan. Add the bacon, onion and garlic and
    fry until the bacon is crisp.
2   Stir in the remaining vegetables (except the kidney beans) and pasta.
    Add seasonings, tomato purée and stock. Bring to boil, stirring con-
    stantly. Reduce the heat, cover and simmer for 20–25 minutes, stirring
    occasionally.

3   Add the kidney beans and simmer for a further 10 minutes or until all the vegetables are tender.
4   Adjust the seasoning to taste before serving and sprinkle with the Parmesan cheese.
5   Serve with bread or rolls.

Tomato Soup

▶ CHO 20g ▶ CALORIES 380 *serves 4*

1 x 15ml sp/1 tbs corn or sunflower oil
1 medium-sized onion, peeled and chopped
2 rashers/slices streaky bacon, rinds removed and chopped
1 x 15ml sp/1 tbs flour
450g/1 lb fresh tomatoes, halved and deseeded
550ml/1 pint/2½ cups chicken stock
salt and freshly ground black pepper
pinch dried basil
lemon juice to taste
1 x 5ml sp/1 tsp intense sweetener

1 Heat the oil in a pan, add the onion and bacon and cook for 5 minutes.
2 Stir in the flour and cook for 1 minute, stirring constantly. Add the tomatoes and gradually stir in the stock.
3 Bring to the boil, then reduce the heat and add the seasonings. Simmer for 20 minutes.
4 Remove the pan from the heat and rub the soup through a sieve. Adjust the seasoning to taste, add lemon juice and sweetener then serve with bread or rolls.

Lentil Soup

▶ CHO 50g ▶ CALORIES 430   *serves 4*

2 onions, peeled and chopped
3 carrots, chopped
100g/4oz/¹/₂ cup lentils
1.1ltr/2 pints/5 cups ham stock
freshly ground black pepper
fresh parsley, to garnish

1   Put the onions, carrots, lentils and stock in a pan.
2   Bring to the boil, then cover and simmer for 40–45 minutes, stirring
    occasionally.
3   Either liquidize the soup or rub it through a sieve. Adjust the seasoning
    to taste, then serve, garnished with parsley, with bread or rolls.

Watercress and Onion Soup

▶ **CHO neg** ▶ **CALORIES 90** *serves 4*

1 bunch watercress, washed and roughly chopped
2 onions, peeled and chopped
550ml/1 pint/2$\frac{1}{2}$ cups vegetable stock
a little grated nutmeg
salt and freshly ground black pepper
a few watercress leaves to garnish

1   Put the watercress and onions in a pan. Add the stock and seasonings.
    Bring to the boil, cover and simmer for 20 minutes.
2   Leave to cool slightly, then pour the soup into a blender or liquidizer
    and blend until smooth.
3   Return the soup to the pan and reheat. Adjust the seasoning to taste.
4   Serve, garnished with the watercress, with bread or rolls.

Turkey or Chicken Broth

▶ **CHO neg** ▶ **CALORIES 200**   *serves 4*

1 chicken or turkey carcass and any leftover meat, diced
3 carrots, peeled and diced
2 leeks, thinly sliced
2 x 15ml sp/2 tbs rice
1 bay leaf
salt and freshly ground black pepper

1   Put the carcass in a large pan and cover with water. Add the remaining
    ingredients and bring to the boil.
2   Reduce the heat and simmer for 2 hours, skimming any froth and fat
    with a spoon when necessary. Add more water if the liquid in the pan
    becomes low.
3   Remove the carcass from the pan. Skim the soup well to remove any
    remaining fat and adjust the seasoning to taste, then serve with bread
    or rolls.

Smoked Mackerel Pâté

▶ **CHO neg** ▶ **CALORIES 800**   *serves 4*

225g/8oz/¹/₂ lb smoked mackerel fillets
100g/4oz/¹/₂ cup skimmed milk soft cheese or low-fat soft cheese
lemon juice to taste
salt and freshly ground black pepper

1   Flake the fish into a bowl. Add the soft cheese and lemon juice and
     season to taste. Mix the ingredients together well by hand or process
     in a liquidizer or blender.
2   Put the pâté into a serving dish and chill until needed.
3   Serve with melba toast.

▶ *Notes to Cooks Will keep in refrigerator for up to 48 hours.*
   Melba toast is light and crisp and can be served instead of rolls with
soup and other appetizers. It is made by cutting bread into thin slices and
toasting slowly in the oven until crisp and golden. Alternatively, it can be
made from thicker slices, toasted on both sides then split through the
middle.

Chicken Liver Pâté

▶ CHO neg ▶ CALORIES 430   *serves 4*

25g/1oz/2 tbs low-fat spread
1 medium onion, finely chopped
225g/8oz/¹⁄₂ lb chicken livers
1 x 5ml sp/1 tsp grated nutmeg
salt and freshly ground black pepper
1 slice lemon

1   Put the low-fat spread in a pan and lightly sauté the onion for 1
    minute. Add the chicken livers and seasonings. Continue cooking for
    5–6 minutes, stirring occasionally. Leave to cool, then liquidize or
    blend until smooth.
2   Put the pâté into the serving dish and smooth the top. Put the lemon
    slice on top. Chill until needed.
3   Serve with melba toast.

▶ *Note to Cooks Will keep in the refrigerator for up to 48 hours.*

Stuffed Pears

▶ CHO 60g ▶ CALORIES 400   *serves 4*

2 dessert pears, cut in half, core removed and sprinkled with lemon
    juice
100g/4oz/$\frac{1}{2}$ cup cottage cheese
25g/1oz/3 tbs walnuts, chopped
1 x 15ml sp/1 tbs raisins
few drops Worcestershire sauce
salt and freshly ground black pepper
lettuce and tomato or lemon slices to garnish

1   Put the pear halves on a lettuce leaf. Put to one side.
2   Meanwhile, put the remaining ingredients in a bowl and mix them
    together well.
3   Pile the mixture into the pear halves and garnish with the tomato or
    lemon slices, then serve immediately.

Guacamole

▶ **CHO neg** ▶ **CALORIES 510**   *serves 4–6*

2 ripe avocados, about 100g/4oz/¼ lb each
1 lemon, juice of
1 small onion, peeled and finely chopped
1 clove garlic, crushed
225g/½ lb tomatoes, skinned, de-seeded and finely chopped
dash of Tabasco sauce
fresh parsley, chopped to garnish

1   Scoop the flesh out from the avocados into a bowl. Mash the lemon juice into the flesh. Add the remaining ingredients and blend well until the mixture is quite smooth.
2   Chill until needed, then transfer it to a serving dish and sprinkle the parsley over it.
3   Serve with a selection of vegetable crudités or tortilla chips.

Mediterranean-style Mackerel

▶ CHO neg ▶ CALORIES 820   *serves 4*

1 x 15ml sp/1 tbs olive oil
1 onion, chopped
1 clove garlic, crushed
1 medium aubergine, cut into small cubes
2 tomatoes, chopped
1 x 5ml sp/1 tsp oregano
1 mackerel, filleted
salt and freshly ground black pepper

1   Heat the oil in a pan and sauté the onions and garlic until tender. Add
    the aubergine and cook for 5 minutes.
2   Add the tomatoes, seasonings and fish and simmer for 20 minutes.
3   Lift out the fish and put it on a serving dish. Serve it topped with the
    vegetables.

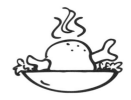

5 meat & poultry

Family meals are often quite a challenge – making food that satisfies everybody's likes and dislikes and doesn't break the budget. We've put together a selection of some family favourites and adapted them so that they are healthier without sacrificing taste.

Inventive use of nourishing economical foods like the cheaper cuts of meat and fish, fresh vegetables in season and dairy products all help to produce delicious inexpensive meals.

Casseroles and stews are tasty, easy to make and to reheat if your family needs to have staggered mealtimes.

Another good idea is to add beans and other pulses to meat dishes. Not only does this increase the fibre but it makes the meat go further.

Stuffed Peppers and Tomatoes

▶ CHO 80g ▶ CALORIES 1570   *serves 4*

4 green peppers
4 large tomatoes
2 x 15ml sp/2 tbs tomato purée diluted in 150ml/$\frac{1}{4}$ pint hot water
1 x 15ml sp/1 tbs corn or sunflower oil

Stuffing

225g/8oz/$\frac{1}{2}$ lb lean, minced beef or lamb
1 large onion, chopped
150ml/$\frac{1}{4}$ pint/3 cups hot water
2 x 15ml sp/2 tbs fresh parsley, finely chopped
salt and freshly ground black pepper
50g/2oz/$\frac{1}{3}$ cup brown rice, cooked
50g/2oz/$\frac{1}{3}$ cup pine kernels
50g/2oz/$\frac{1}{3}$ cup sultanas

1   Cut a slice off the top of each pepper and tomato and reserve them.
    Deseed the peppers. Scoop out most of the tomato flesh, chop it and
    reserve it for the stuffing.
2   To make the stuffing, cook the meat and onions in a pan until they
    brown. Add the hot water, the reserved tomato flesh and seasoning
    ingredients. Mix well and cook for 15 minutes. Add the remaining
    ingredients, mix well and cook for 3 minutes. Arrange the tomatoes
    and peppers upright in a baking dish. Fill them with the stuffing, leav-
    ing a little room for it to expand and replace the reserved tops.

3 Pour the tomato purée mixture over them and cook at 375°F/190°C/ gas mark 5 for 1 hour and 10 minutes, basting them occasionally. If all the liquid evaporates, add a few tablespoons of water.

Broccoli in Ham and Cheese Sauce

▶ CHO 30g ▶ CALORIES 540   *serves 2*

225g/8oz/¹/₂ lb broccoli, cut into even-sized pieces
25g/1oz/2 tbs low-fat spread
25g/1oz/¹/₄ cup wholemeal flour
275ml/¹/₂ pint/3³/₄ cups skimmed milk
50g/2oz/¹/₂ cup reduced-fat cheddar cheese, grated
50g/2oz/4 tbs lean ham, finely chopped
1 x 5ml sp/1 tsp wholegrain mustard
salt and freshly ground black pepper

1   Cook the broccoli until just tender but still crisp. Meanwhile, make the
     sauce.
2   Melt the low-fat spread over a low heat, add the flour and stir over the
     heat for 1 minute. Gradually add the milk, stirring, and bring to the
     boil. Reduce the heat and simmer for about 3 minutes. Reserve a
     tablespoon of the cheese and stir the remainder into the sauce. Stir in
     the ham, mustard and seasoning.
3   Arrange the broccoli in an ovenproof dish, pour the cheese sauce over
     it and sprinkle the reserved cheese over the top. Grill until the grated
     cheese melts and turns golden brown. Serve immediately with pota-
     toes or bread.

Pork Stir-Fry

▶ CHO neg ▶ CALORIES 790   *serves 4*

1 x 15ml sp/1 tbs olive or sunflower oil
350g/12oz/³/₄ lb lean pork tenderloin fillet, cut into thin strips
2.5cm/1 inch root ginger, peeled and finely chopped
1 carrot, peeled and diced
1 onion, peeled and finely chopped
2 small courgettes, washed and sliced
100g/4oz/²/₃ cup baby sweetcorn
225g/8oz/4 cups beansprouts
2 x 15ml sp/2 tbs dry sherry
2 x 15ml sp/2 tbs light soy sauce
freshly ground black pepper

1   Heat the oil in a wok or large frying pan. Add the pork, ginger and onion and stir-fry for 5 to 10 minutes or until the pork is cooked.
2   Add the carrot, onion, courgettes and corn and stir-fry for 5 to 10 minutes. Stir in the beansprouts, sherry and soy sauce. Mix well and stir-fry for 1 minute.
3   Season to taste with freshly ground black pepper and serve immediately with steamed rice or noodles.

Sweet-and-Sour Chicken

▶ CHO 30g ▶ CALORIES 760 *serves 4*

1 x 15ml sp/1 tbs olive or sunflower oil
3 boneless chicken breasts, skin removed, diced
1 onion, sliced
1 green pepper, deseeded and chopped
1 red pepper, deseeded and chopped
225g/1 x 8oz can/1 cup tomatoes
225g/1 x 8oz can/$1^{1}/_{2}$ cups pineapple pieces in natural juice
1 x 15ml sp/1 tbs vinegar
1 x 15ml sp/1 tbs soy sauce
about 150ml/$^{1}/_{4}$ pint/$^{2}/_{3}$ cup water
salt and freshly ground black pepper

1   Heat the oil and lightly fry the chicken and onion for 5 minutes. Add
    the remaining ingredients.
2   Bring to the boil, stirring, cover and simmer for 20–30 minutes or until
    the chicken is tender, adding a little more water if it starts to get a bit
    dry.
3   Serve with rice and vegetable stir-fry.

Stir-Fried Chicken with Cashews

▶ CHO 30g ▶ CALORIES 1090   *serves 4*

4 boneless, skinless chicken breasts, cut into even-sized pieces
2.5cm/1 inch piece root ginger, peeled and chopped
2–3 cloves garlic, crushed
1–2 x 5ml sp/1–2 tsp cornflour
1 x 15ml sp/1 tbs dry sherry
1 x 15ml sp/1 tbs light soy sauce
150ml/¼ pint/⅔ cup chicken stock
1 x 15ml sp/1 tbs olive or sunflower oil
50g/2oz/3½ tbs unsalted cashew nuts
salt and freshly ground black pepper

1 Put the chicken, ginger and garlic in a bowl and leave to stand. Meanwhile, mix the cornflour with the sherry, soy sauce and chicken stock.

2 Heat the oil in a large frying pan or wok. Add the nuts and stir-fry until they are lightly browned. Remove them, then add the chicken, ginger and garlic and stir-fry until the chicken is cooked and tender.

3 Add the sherry, soy sauce and stock mixture and stir until the liquid has thickened. If the sauce becomes too thick, add a little water.

4 Season to taste with salt and freshly ground black pepper. Add the cashew nuts, mix them in well, heat it through, then serve immediately with vegetables and rice or noodles.

Lemon and Herb Baked Chicken

▶ **CHO neg** ▶ **CALORIES 370**   *serves 2*

2 skinless, boned chicken breasts
½ lemon, juice of
2 x 5ml sp/2 tsp olive or sunflower oil
1 clove garlic, crushed
freshly ground black pepper
pinch mixed herbs

1   Score the chicken breasts with a sharp knife and lay them in an oven-proof dish.
2   In a small bowl, mix the lemon juice, oil, garlic, pepper and herbs.
3   Spoon the mixture over the chicken, leave to marinate for 30 minutes. Then bake at 375°F/190°C/gas mark 5 for 30 minutes, until the chicken is cooked.
4   Serve with new potatoes and vegetables.

Chicken Breasts with Pineapple Sauce

▶ CHO 40g ▶ CALORIES 900   *serves 4*

1 x 220g/8oz can/1½ cups pineapple slices in natural juice
1 x 15ml sp/1 tbs olive or sunflower oil
4 boneless, skinless chicken breasts
1 onion, sliced
1 garlic clove, crushed
½ green pepper, deseeded and cut into strips
½ red pepper, deseeded and cut into strips
1–2 x 15ml sp/1–2 tbs wine vinegar
3 x 15ml sp/3 tbs tomato purée
275ml/½ pint/3¾ cups chicken stock
salt and freshly ground black pepper

1   Drain and cube the pineapple, reserving 4 tablespoons of juice.
2   Heat the oil over a moderate heat in a large saucepan, add the chicken and seal on all sides. Remove with a slotted spoon, drain on kitchen paper and set aside.
3   Stir-fry the onion, garlic and pepper in the remaining oil for 2 minutes. Remove the vegetables with a slotted spoon and set aside.
4   Boil the vinegar in the pan until reduced to half the quantity. Stir in tomato purée and stock, return to the boil. Add the reserved pine-apple juice, chicken and vegetables.
5   Season to taste, cover and simmer for 35 minutes or until chicken is cooked. If necessary adjust the seasoning, stir in the pineapple chunks, cover and cook for a further 10 minutes.
6   Serve with broccoli florets and vegetable rice (see page 158).

Greek-Style Lamb Kebabs

▶ **CHO neg** ▶ **CALORIES 1820** *serves 4–6*

2 x 15ml sp/2 tbs corn or sunflower oil
½ lemon, juice of
1–2 cloves of garlic, crushed
675g/1½ lb boned leg of lamb, cut into cubes
salt
cayenne pepper

1 Beat the oil, lemon juice and garlic together and let the meat marinate in it for 4 hours, covered in a refrigerator, basting the meat occasionally.
2 Thread the meat onto skewers and grill for 8–10 minutes, turning the skewers to brown the meat on all sides. Brush the kebabs with the marinade once or twice. Allow an extra 5 minutes if cooking on a barbecue.
3 Season with salt and cayenne pepper to taste and serve immediately with salad and rice or pitta bread.

Minced Beef Cobbler

▶ CHO 80g ▶ CALORIES 1140   *serves 4*

450g/1 lb extra lean minced beef
1 onion, peeled and chopped
2 carrots, peeled and diced
227g/1 x 8oz can/1 cup tomatoes
about 150ml/¼ pint/⅔ cup beef stock
salt and freshly ground black pepper

Cobbler

100g/4oz/1 cup fine self-raising wholemeal flour
1 x 5ml sp/1 tsp baking powder
pinch salt
25g/1oz/2 tbs low-fat spread
150ml/¼ pint/⅔ cup skimmed milk

1   Sauté the mince, onion and carrots in a saucepan until the mince is all lightly browned. Add the tomatoes and stock and simmer for 30 minutes, stirring occasionally. Season to taste with salt and freshly ground black pepper.

2   Meanwhile, rub the fat into the flour, baking powder and salt until the mixture resembles fine breadcrumbs, then stir in enough milk to form a soft dough. Roll it out on a lightly floured surface until it is 1cm (½ inch) thick and, using a 5cm (2 inch) cutter, cut out circles.

3   Pour the mince mixture into an ovenproof dish and place the dough 'cobbles' around the edge, overlapping them. Brush them with the remaining milk and bake at 400°F/200°C/gas mark 6 for 10–12 minutes, until the cobbler has risen and turned golden brown. Serve immediately with peas and mashed potatoes, giving everyone a serving of the cobbler with their savoury mince.

Beefburger Surprise

▶ **CHO neg** ▶ **CALORIES 700** *serves 4*

450g/1 lb extra lean minced beef
1 onion, peeled and finely chopped
salt and freshly ground black pepper
50g/2oz/¹⁄₂ cup reduced-fat cheddar cheese, grated

1 Put the mince, onion and seasonings into a bowl and mix them together well. Divide the mixture in half and shape each into an 18cm (7 inch) round. Sprinkle the cheese evenly over one round to within 1cm (¹⁄₂ inch) of the edges. Cover the cheese layer with the second round and pinch the edges together firmly, sealing the filling inside.

2 Cook the burger under the grill for approximately 6–8 minutes each side, or until cooked through. Cut it into quarters and serve in a brown roll with salad.

Cottage Pie

▶ **CHO 100g** ▶ **CALORIES 1190**   *serves 4–6*

450g/1 lb extra lean minced beef
1 onion, peeled and chopped
2 carrots, peeled and finely chopped
227g/1 x 8oz can/1 cup tomatoes
1 x 15ml sp/1 tbs tomato purée
about 150ml/$^1/_4$ pint/$^2/_3$ cup beef stock
salt and freshly ground black pepper
600g/22oz/2$^3/_4$ cups potatoes, peeled, boiled and mashed

1   Sauté the minced beef, onions and carrots until the meat is all just
     brown, stirring occasionally. Stir in the tomatoes, tomato purée and
     stock. Season to taste with salt and freshly ground black pepper, cover
     and simmer for 30 minutes.

2   Spoon the mixture into an ovenproof dish and spread the mashed
     potato over the meat. Decorate the surface of the potato by drawing
     wavy lines on it with a fork.

3   Bake the pie in the oven at 375°F/190°C/gas mark 5 for 30–35 min-
     utes. If liked, place the pie under the grill just before serving to brown
     the potato topping.

4   Serve with vegetables.

Macaroni Mince

▶ CHO 50g ▶ CALORIES 1130   *serves 4*

450g/1 lb extra lean minced beef
2 medium onions, finely chopped
1 clove garlic, crushed
1 medium carrot, finely diced
227g/1 x 8oz can/1 cup tomatoes
salt and freshly ground black pepper
pinch mixed herbs
about 150ml/$\frac{1}{4}$ pint/$\frac{2}{3}$ cup beef stock
225g/8oz/4 cups macaroni, cooked
50g/2oz/$\frac{1}{2}$ cup half-fat hard cheese, grated

1   Put the mince, onion, garlic and carrot in a pan and fry gently until all
     the mince has browned, stirring occasionally. Stir in the remaining
     ingredients and seasonings except the macaroni and cheese, bring to
     the boil and simmer for 20 minutes.
2   Once cooked, pour the macaroni into an ovenproof dish, put the
     mince over the macaroni and top with the grated cheese. Melt the
     cheese under the grill, then serve hot with vegetables or salad.

Spaghetti Bolognese

▶ **CHO neg** ▶ **CALORIES 560**   *serves 4*

350g/12oz/³/₄ cup extra lean minced beef
1 onion, finely chopped
1 clove garlic, crushed
2 carrots, finely chopped
2 sticks celery, thinly sliced
100g/4oz/1¹/₂ cups mushrooms, sliced
400g/1 x 14oz can/1³/₄ cups tomatoes, chopped, with juice
1 x 15ml sp/1 tbs tomato purée
150ml/¹/₄ pint/²/₃ cup beef stock
1 x 2.5ml sp/¹/₂ tsp basil
1 x 2.5ml sp/¹/₂ tsp oregano
salt and freshly ground black pepper

1   Brown the minced beef in a large pan without added fat for 5 minutes.
     Drain off any excess fat, then add the onion, garlic, carrot, celery and
     mushrooms and stir well. Add the remaining ingredients and season to
     taste with salt and freshly ground black pepper. Bring to the boil and
     simmer gently for 30–40 minutes, stirring occasionally.
2   While the Bolognese sauce is cooking, bring a large pan of salted
     water to the boil and cook the spaghetti. When the spaghetti is *al
     dente* and the Bolognese sauce is ready, drain the spaghetti and either
     add it to the sauce and mix well together or serve a nest of spaghetti
     on each plate, topped with the Bolognese sauce.

▶ *Note to Cooks Remember to take into account the CHO values of any
spaghetti. 45g cooked weight of wholemeal spaghetti = 10g CHO.*

Moussaka

▶ CHO 140g ▶ CALORIES 1600   *serves 4–6*

1 large aubergine (about 275g/10oz), sliced and sprinkled
   with 1 tsp salt
1 x 15ml sp/1 tbs corn or sunflower oil
450g/1 lb extra lean minced lamb
1 large onion, chopped
1 clove garlic, crushed
1 x 5ml sp/1 tsp cinnamon
2 x 15ml sp/2 tbs fresh parsley, chopped
salt and freshly ground black pepper
3 x 15ml sp/3 tbs tomato purée
600g/22oz/3 cups potatoes, parboiled and sliced

White sauce

25g/1oz/2 tbs low-fat spread
25g/1oz/^{1}/4 cup flour
275ml/^{1}/2 pint/3^3/4 cups skimmed milk
salt and freshly ground black pepper
pinch ground nutmeg
1 egg yolk

1   Once the aubergines have rendered their bitter juices, pat them dry
    with absorbent kitchen paper. Heat the oil in a large frying pan and fry
    the aubergine slices until they are golden brown on both sides. Drain
    them on absorbent kitchen paper.
2   Meanwhile, sauté the lamb, onion and garlic until all the meat is
    brown. Add the cinnamon, parsley, salt and pepper to taste, tomato
    purée and a little water to moisten.

3   In a large, ovenproof casserole, put alternate layers of potatoes, meat and aubergines starting and ending with a potato layer.

4   Make the white sauce and allow it to cool slightly before mixing in the egg yolk. Spoon the sauce over the potatoes in the dish and bake at 375°F/190°C/gas mark 5 for 25–30 minutes or until the top is golden brown.

Navarin of Lamb

▶ CHO 10g ▶ CALORIES 1150   *serves 4*

1 x 15ml sp/1 tbs corn or sunflower oil
1 large onion, chopped
1 clove garlic, crushed
4 chump chops, trimmed of fat
1 x 15ml sp/1 tbs flour
2 carrots, sliced
1 small, swede (about 225g/$\frac{1}{2}$ lb), peeled and chopped
1 x 15ml sp/1 tbs tomato purée
400g/1 x 14oz can/$1\frac{3}{4}$ cups chopped tomatoes
1 bouquet garni
freshly ground black pepper
fresh parsley, chopped, to garnish

1   Heat the oil in a flameproof casserole. Add the onion and garlic and fry for 5 minutes.
2   Meanwhile, coat the lamb chops in the flour. Add them to the casserole and brown them quickly on both sides. Add the carrots, swede, tomato purée and tomatoes and bring to the boil.
3   Add the seasonings. Cover with a lid and transfer to oven and cook at 325°F/170°C/gas mark 3 for 1–2 hours, until the meat is tender. Adjust the seasoning to taste and sprinkle the chopped parsley over before serving with new potatoes or rice, plus vegetables.

Beef Stew and Dumplings

▶ CHO 100g ▶ CALORIES 2430   *serves 4*

2 x 15ml sp/2 tbs corn or sunflower oil
675g/1½ lb braising steak, trimmed and cut into cubes
3 sticks celery, sliced
3 small carrots, peeled and sliced
1 small swede (about 100g/4oz), peeled and cubed
2 onions, peeled and chopped
2 x 15ml sp/2 tbs flour
2 x 15ml sp/2 tbs tomato purée
500ml/1 pint/2½ cups beef stock
2 bay leaves
freshly ground black pepper

Dumpling mixture

100g/4oz/1 cup self-raising wholemeal flour
50g/2oz/⅓ cup vegetable suet
pinch salt
1 x 15ml sp/1 tbs parsley, chopped
sufficient water to bind

1   Heat the oil in a large, flameproof casserole. Add the meat and fry until it has browned to seal in the flavour (about 5 minutes). Add all the prepared vegetables and fry for 3 minutes. Stir in the flour and cook for 1 minute, stirring. Stir in the tomato purée, stock, bay leaves and seasoning and bring to the boil. Cover with the lid and bake at 350°F/180°C/gas mark 4 for 1–2 hours, until the meat is tender.

2 To make the dumplings, sift the flour into a bowl and stir in the suet, seasoning and parsley. Mix to a firm (not sticky) dough with water (about 5 tbs). Form into 8 dumplings and put them on top of the meat in the casserole for the last 20 minutes or so until the dumplings are light and fluffy (do not remove the lid during this 20 minutes).

Carbonade of Beef

▶ CHO 10g ▶ CALORIES 1640   *serves 4*

2 x 15ml sp/2 tbs corn or sunflower oil
675g/1½ lb chuck steak, cut into cubes
1 onion, peeled and chopped
4 celery stalks, chopped
2 carrots, sliced
1 x 15ml sp/1 tbs flour
salt and freshly ground black pepper
1 x 5ml sp/1 tsp vinegar
1 bouquet garni
275ml/½ pint/1⅓ cups stout
fresh parsley, chopped, to garnish

1   Heat the oil in a flameproof casserole, then add the cubes of meat and
    brown them quickly on all sides. Add the vegetables and cook for 5
    minutes. Stir in flour, seasonings, vinegar, bouquet garni and stout.
2   Cover the casserole and bake at 325°F/170°C/gas mark 3 for 1–2
    hours, or until the meat is tender. Stir a little water into the casserole if
    it becomes dry during the cooking time.
3   Discard the bouquet garni and adjust the seasoning to taste just
    before serving with potatoes or bread.

Barbecued Pork Chops

▶ CHO neg ▶ CALORIES 430   *serves 2*

2 lean pork chops or pork steaks

Barbecue sauce

1 x 15ml sp/1 tbs chilli sauce
1 x 15ml sp/1 tbs Worcestershire sauce
1 x 15ml sp/1 tbs vinegar
1 x 15ml sp/1 tbs tomato ketchup
1 x 5ml sp/1 tsp light soy sauce
1 clove garlic, crushed

1   Mix the barbecue sauce ingredients together.
2   Put the chops or steaks in a casserole dish and bake at 375°F/190°C/
     gas mark 5 for approximately 10–15 minutes or until the chops are
     browned. Pour off any fat. Pour the sauce over them and re-cover.
     Bake for 25–30 more minutes, basting them occasionally.
3   Arrange them on a serving dish and spoon the sauce over them.
4   Serve with jacket potato and salad or rice and vegetables.

6 fish

There are two main types of fish: the oily ones – such as mackerel – and white fish – such as cod, haddock and so on. The oils in oily fish are excellent sources of vitamins A and D and are also thought to protect the body against heart disease.

    With the recipes in this chapter for both white and oily fish, you can cook up a tempting feast that will also benefit your general well-being.

Tuna Sauce

▶ CHO 70g ▶ CALORIES 660 *serves 3–4*

1 x 15ml sp/1 tbs olive oil
2 cloves garlic, crushed
2–3 sticks celery, chopped
1 bay leaf
pinch oregano
salt and freshly ground black pepper
200g/1 x 7oz can/$^3/_4$ cup tuna fish in brine, drained and flaked
400g/1 x 14oz can/1$^3/_4$ cups tomatoes
3 x 15ml sp/3 tbs tomato purée

1 Heat the oil in a pan and fry the garlic and celery. Add the herbs and seasoning to taste with salt and freshly ground black pepper. Stir in the tuna fish, tomatoes and tomato purée. Bring to the boil and simmer gently for 20–30 minutes.
2 Meanwhile cook the pasta in plenty of boiling salted water. Serve the tuna sauce as soon as it is ready on a bed of *al dente* pasta accompanied by salad.

▶ *Note to Cooks Remember to take into account the CHO values of any spaghetti: 45g cooked weight of wholemeal spaghetti = 10g CHO.*

Baked Fish

▶ CHO 10g ▶ CALORIES 850   *serves 4*

4 cod steaks
3 x 15ml sp/3 tbs olive or sunflower oil
2 cloves garlic, finely sliced
4 x 15ml sp/4 tbs fresh parsley, finely chopped
450g/1 lb tomatoes, deseeded and finely chopped
salt and freshly ground black pepper
2 x 15ml sp/2 tbs wholemeal breadcrumbs, toasted

1   Arrange the fish in a lightly oiled baking dish.
2   Meanwhile, lightly beat together all other ingredients, apart from the
    breadcrumbs. Spread some of the mixture over each slice of fish,
    sprinkle with the breadcrumbs and bake at 375°F/190°C/gas mark 5
    for 30–40 minutes, basting occasionally, until crisp on top.
3   Serve with julienne vegetables and new potatoes.

Smoked Haddock Plait

▶ CHO 110g ▶ CALORIES 1380   *serves 4–6*

25g/1oz/2 tbs low-fat spread
1 onion, peeled and chopped
25g/1oz/¼ cup flour
275ml/½ pint/1⅓ cups skimmed milk
salt and freshly ground black pepper
1 x 15ml sp/1 tbs lemon juice
225g/8oz/1 cup smoked haddock, cooked and flaked
50g/2oz/⅓ cup sweetcorn
215g/7oz/½ lb puff pastry
1 hard-boiled egg, sliced
a little beaten egg to glaze

1   Heat the low-fat spread in a pan and sauté the onion. Add the flour
    and milk and stir continuously, until the sauce has thickened. Season to
    taste with salt and freshly ground black pepper. Add the lemon juice,
    fish and sweetcorn.
2   Roll the pastry out into an oblong shape 20 by 30cm (8 by 12 inches)
    and spoon the filling down the centre third of the pastry, layering it
    with the eggs.
3   Cut the pastry diagonally at 2cm (1 inch) intervals down each side
    of the oblong. Fold down the top and take one strip from each side of
    the pastry and cross them over the fish. Continue in this way to form a
    plait. Brush with the beaten egg and bake at 400°F/200°C/ gas mark 6
    for approximately 25 minutes, or until the pastry is golden brown.
4   Serve with salad.

Prawn and Cashew Nut Curry

▶ CHO 20g ▶ CALORIES 930   *serves 4*

1 x 15ml sp/1 tbs corn or sunflower oil
1 large onion, peeled and chopped
1–2 cloves garlic, crushed
1.5cm/^{1}/$_2$ inch piece fresh root ginger, peeled and finely chopped
2 x 5ml sp/2 tsp ground coriander
2 x 5ml sp/2 tsp paprika
2 x 5ml sp/2 tsp ground cumin
400g/1 x 14oz can/1^3/$_4$ cups chopped tomatoes
350g/12oz/3 cups frozen prawns, thawed
50g/2oz/3^1/$_2$ tbs unsalted cashew nuts, lightly toasted and chopped
150g/1 x 5fl oz carton/^{2}/$_3$ cup low-fat natural yogurt
salt and freshly ground black pepper

1   Heat the oil in a pan and gently fry the onion, garlic and ginger. Add
    the spices and fry for about a minute.
2   Add the chopped tomatoes, prawns and nuts and stir together well.
    Stir in the yogurt and seasonings and heat gently for about 5 minutes.
    Serve immediately with rice.

▶ *Note to Cooks Remember to take into account the CHO values of any
rice – 3 tbs/3 x 15ml spoonfuls = 10g CHO.*

Paprika Fish

▶ CHO 40g ▶ CALORIES 920   *serves 4*

1 x 15ml sp/1 tbs corn or sunflower oil
2 onions, peeled and sliced
2 medium-size potatoes, peeled and cut into 2cm/³⁄₄ inch dice
1 green pepper, deseeded and cut into strips
1 red pepper, deseeded and cut into strips
1–2 x 15ml sp/1–2 tbs paprika
salt and freshly ground black pepper
about 210ml/7fl oz/³⁄₄ cup water
675g/1¹⁄₂ lb haddock fillet, cut into strips

1   Heat the oil in a pan, add the onion and potato and cook over a low
    heat, stirring frequently, for 5 minutes. Add the peppers and paprika
    and season with salt and freshly ground black pepper. Mix in the water
    and simmer over a low heat for approximately 20 minutes until the
    vegetables are tender.
2   Add the fish and simmer for a further 5–6 minutes until the fish is just
    cooked. Serve immediately with more potatoes and vegetables.

Fish-Stuffed Baked Potatoes

▶ CHO 230g ▶ CALORIES 1170   *serves 4*

4 medium-sized baking potatoes, washed
225g/8oz/^{1}/$_2$ lb white fish
100g/4oz/^{1}/$_2$ cup skimmed-milk cheese or low-fat cheese
1 clove garlic, crushed
1 x 15ml sp/1 tbs fresh chives, finely chopped
salt and freshly ground black pepper

1   Bake the potatoes at 400°F/200°C/gas mark 6 for approximately 1
    hour or until potatoes are tender.
2   Meanwhile, steam the fish for about 6 minutes until just tender and
    flake it into a bowl, removing any bones and skin. When the potatoes
    are cooked, cut a slice off the top of each potato and scoop out the
    flesh into a bowl. Mash it with the cheese and garlic. Fold in the fish
    and chives and season to taste with salt and freshly ground black
    pepper.
3   Fill each potato shell with the mixture and bake them at 350°F/180°C/
    gas mark 4 for 10–15 minutes or until the filling has heated through.
    Serve immediately with salad.

Mackerel with Lime

▶ CHO neg ▶ CALORIES 2060   *serves 4*

4 mackerel (each about 225g/8oz), gutted and filleted
2 limes, peeled and sliced
bunch spring onions, chopped
salt and freshly ground black pepper
150ml/$^1/_4$ pint/$^2/_3$ cup dry cider
2 bay leaves

1   Put the mackerel in a lightly greased baking dish. Arrange the lime slices and spring onions down the middle of each fish and season with salt and freshly ground black pepper. Close each fish up and secure with wooden cocktail sticks. Pour the cider over them and add the bay leaves.
2   Cover and cook at 350°F/180°C/gas mark 4 for 30–40 minutes or until tender. Serve hot with vegetables and potatoes.

Kedgeree

▶ CHO 70g ▶ CALORIES 1170   *serves 4*

450g/1 lb smoked haddock
150ml/¼ pint/⅔ cup skimmed milk
175g/6oz/1 cup brown rice, cooked
2 size 3 eggs, hard-boiled
175g/6oz/1 cup frozen peas, cooked
salt and freshly ground black pepper
fresh parsley, chopped, to garnish

1   Poach the fish in the milk for 10–12 minutes or until tender. Drain, reserving the liquor. Remove any skin from the fish and flake the flesh.

2   Add the fish and rice to a pan. Stir in the egg, and a little of the fish liquor. Add peas and season to taste with salt and freshly ground black pepper, then cook gently over a low heat until heated through.

3   Serve immediately, garnished with the parsley.

Sailor's Pie

1 x 15ml sp/1 tbs corn or sunflower oil
1 onion, peeled and sliced
2 sticks celery, sliced
50g/2oz/³⁄₄ cup button mushrooms, sliced
3 tomatoes, sliced
salt and freshly ground black pepper
350g/12oz/2 cups white fish, cooked and flaked
2–3 drops Tabasco sauce
225g/8oz/3 cups potatoes, parboiled and sliced

1   Heat the oil in a pan and sauté the onion and celery for 2–3 minutes. Add the mushrooms and tomatoes and cook for 3–4 minutes. Put half the mixture in an ovenproof casserole.

2   Season the fish to taste with salt and freshly ground black pepper and put it into the casserole, mixing it in together with the Tabasco sauce. Top with the remaining vegetables.

3   Arrange the sliced potatoes in overlapping circles on top of the casserole and lay a piece of dampened greaseproof paper over them. Cover with foil and bake at 350°F/180°C/gas mark 4 for approximately 1 hour. Then remove the foil and paper and cook under a grill for 2–3 minutes to brown the potatoes. Serve immediately.

Haddock Crumble

▶ CHO 100g ▶ CALORIES 1100   *serves 4*

450g/1 lb haddock
275ml/^{1}/₂ pint/1^1/₃ cups skimmed milk
1 x 15ml sp/1 tbs corn or sunflower oil
1 onion, peeled and chopped
2 x 5ml sp/2 tsp curry powder
25g/1oz/^{1}/₄ cup flour
1 x 15ml sp//1 tbs sultanas
1 x 15ml sp/1 tbs mango chutney
50g/2oz/^{1}/₃ cup frozen sweetcorn, cooked
salt and freshly ground black pepper

Crumble topping
25g/1oz/^{1}/₄ cup porridge oats
25g/1oz/^{1}/₄ cup wholemeal flour
25g/1oz/2 tbs low-fat spread
1 x 15ml sp/1 tbs fresh parsley, chopped
salt and freshly ground black pepper

1   Put the fish and milk in a pan and poach for 10–15 minutes, then drain off the liquid and reserve it. Flake the fish, removing any bones or skin, and put it in a lightly greased ovenproof dish.

2   Heat the oil in a pan and sauté the onion. Stir in the curry powder and flour and cook, stirring, for 1 minute. Stir in the milk and bring to the boil, stirring until it is thick and smooth. Add the sultanas, chutney and sweetcorn. Season to taste with salt and freshly ground black pepper, then pour the sauce over the fish.

3   To make the topping, put the oats and flour in a bowl. Rub in the low-fat spread, then stir in the parsley and seasoning. Spoon it evenly over the fish and cook in the oven at 350°F/180°C/gas mark 4 for 40 minutes. Serve immediately.

Steamed Trout with Yogurt Sauce

▶ CHO 10g ▶ CALORIES 750   *serves 4*

4 trout (each about 175g/6oz), gutted and cleaned
4 x 15ml sp/4 tbs lemon juice
1 x 15ml sp/1 tbs fresh parsley, chopped
freshly ground black pepper

Yogurt sauce

1 x 150g/5fl oz carton/$^2/_3$ cup low-fat natural yogurt
1 x 15ml sp/1 tbs horseradish sauce
2 x 15ml sp/2 tbs lemon juice
1–2 x 5ml sp/1–2 tsp fresh chives, chopped
pinch cayenne pepper

1   Put the trout on a large sheet of foil and season with the lemon juice, parsley and pepper. Fold the foil loosely round the fish to form a parcel and steam for 10 to 15 minutes, or until fish flakes easily when tested with a fork.

2   Meanwhile, to make the sauce, put all the ingredients in a heatproof bowl. Put it over a pan of simmering water and stir until it is hot and creamy. Remove the trout from the boil and serve immediately with the yogurt sauce poured over them accompanied by julienne vegetables and new potatoes.

Stuffed Plaice

▶ CHO 40g ▶ CALORIES 1450　　　　　*serves 4*

8 medium plaice fillets, skinned
3 x 15ml sp/3 tbs unsweetened apple juice
1 x 15ml sp/1 tbs soy sauce

Stuffing

50g/2oz/1 cup fresh wholemeal breadcrumbs
1–2 cloves garlic, crushed
1 small onion, peeled and finely chopped
25g/1oz/$\frac{1}{4}$ cup ground almonds
1 x 2.5ml sp/$\frac{1}{2}$ tsp ground ginger
2 x 15ml sp/2 tbs unsweetened apple juice
1 x 15ml sp/1 tbs soy sauce
freshly ground black pepper

1　Lay the fillets flesh-side down on a clean surface.
2　To make the stuffing, put all the ingredients in a bowl and mix them
　　together well. Divide the stuffing between the fillets and roll up, secur-
　　ing them with cocktail sticks. Put the rolls in a shallow, lightly greased
　　ovenproof dish.
3　Mix together the apple juice and soy sauce and pour this over the
　　rolled fish. Cover with foil and cook at 350°F/180°C/gas mark 4 for 30
　　minutes. Serve immediately with vegetables and new potatoes.

Haddock and Vegetable Casserole

▶ CHO 40g ▶ CALORIES 720   *serves 4*

1 x 15ml sp/1 tbs corn or sunflower oil
1 onion, peeled and sliced
1 green pepper, deseeded and chopped
3 tomatoes, chopped
1 x 5ml sp/1 tsp oregano
225g/8oz/1⅓ cups potatoes, peeled and cubed
1 x 15ml sp/1 tbs tomato purée
salt and freshly ground black pepper
450g/1 lb haddock fillet, skinned and cut into large pieces
3 x 15ml sp/3 tbs lemon juice
2 courgettes, sliced

1   Heat the oil in a pan and sauté the onion and pepper for 2–3 minutes.
    Add the tomatoes, oregano, potatoes, tomato purée and season to
    taste with salt and freshly ground black pepper. Bring to the boil, cover
    and simmer for 20 minutes, until the potatoes are just tender.
2   Meanwhile, put the fish and lemon juice in a bowl and season. Mix
    them together well, then add them to the pan, along with the cour-
    gettes, cover and simmer for 10 minutes until the fish is tender. Serve
    immediately with jacket potatoes.

Baked Fish with Pepper Sauce

▶ CHO neg ▶ CALORIES 1070

serves 4

4 cod or haddock fillets (each about 175g/6oz)
25g/1oz/2 tbs low-fat spread, melted
4 x 15ml sp/4 tbs lemon juice
salt and freshly ground black pepper

Pepper sauce

1 x 15ml sp/1 tbs corn or sunflower oil
2 red peppers, deseeded and chopped
1 small onion, peeled and chopped
2 x 15ml sp/2 tbs half-fat crème fraiche
lemon twists to garnish

1   Put the fish in a lightly greased baking dish and brush with the melted low-fat spread. Drizzle with the lemon juice and season to taste with salt and freshly ground black pepper. Cover with foil and cook at 350°F/180°C/gas mark 4 for 20–25 minutes, until tender.
2   Meanwhile, make the sauce. Heat the oil, add the pepper and onion and cook for 5 minutes. Add 3 tbs of water, bring to the boil, cover and cook gently for 10–15 minutes. Transfer the sauce to a blender and process until smooth. Return it to the pan, stir in the crème fraiche and season to taste. Reheat it gently, then serve the fish on warmed serving plates and with the sauce, garnished with the lemon twists and accompanied by vegetables and potatoes.

Rice with Prawns

▶ CHO 140g ▶ CALORIES 1110   *serves 6*

2 x 15ml sp/2 tbs corn or sunflower oil
1 onion, peeled and chopped
1 clove garlic, crushed
1 x 5ml sp/1 tsp ground coriander
1 x 5ml sp/1 tsp ground cumin
1 x 5ml sp/1 tsp curry powder
175g/6oz/1½ cups frozen prawns, thawed
1 x 15ml sp/1 tbs soy sauce
100g/4oz/⅔ cup frozen peas, cooked
salt and freshly ground black pepper
175g/6oz/1 cup brown rice, cooked
3 spring onions, chopped

1   Heat the oil, add the onion and garlic and fry until they have softened.
    Add the coriander, cumin and curry powder and stir until they are well
    combined. Stir in the prawns until they are coated in the spices. Add
    the soy sauce, peas, 4 tbs of water and season to taste with salt and
    freshly ground black pepper. Cook the mixture for 2 minutes, then add
    the rice and mix everything together thoroughly. Cover and cook
    gently until it has heated through.
2   Turn the mixture onto a warmed serving dish, sprinkle the spring
    onions over it and serve immediately.

Mackerel with Mustard and Oats

▶ CHO 10g ▶ CALORIES 1650 *serves 4*

4 mackerel fillets (each about 175g/6oz)
1 x 15ml sp/1 tbs lemon juice
salt and freshly ground black pepper
2 x 5ml sp/2 tsp made mustard
25g/1oz/¼ cup porridge oats

1 Put the mackerel on a grill rack lined with foil. Drizzle the lemon juice over the fish and season with salt and freshly ground black pepper.
2 Stir the mustard and oats together and spread the mixture over the mackerel. Cook the fish under a medium-hot grill for 10–15 minutes, then serve immediately with vegetables and potatoes.

Fish Creole

▶ CHO neg ▶ CALORIES 560   *serves 4*

1 onion, peeled and chopped
1 green pepper, deseeded and chopped
1 x 400g/14oz can/1¾ cups chopped tomatoes
pinch basil
pinch oregano
salt and freshly ground black pepper
225g/8oz/1⅓ cups white fish, cut into cubes
225g/8oz/2 cups frozen prawns, defrosted
1 x 5ml sp/1 tsp cornflour
2 x 15ml sp/2 tbs dry white wine
fresh parsley, chopped, to garnish

1   Put the onion, pepper, tomatoes and herbs and seasoning in a pan
    and bring to the boil. Cover and simmer for 10 minutes. Add the fish
    and prawns and simmer for a further 10–15 minutes.
2   Blend the cornflour with the wine, then stir this mixture into the sauce
    and stir for 1–2 minutes while it thickens. Serve immediately, garnished
    with the chopped parsley, accompanied by vegetables and potatoes.

Fish Steaks and Peppercorn Sauce

▶ CHO 30g ▶ CALORIES 940   *serves 6*

6 white fish steaks or cutlets
25g/1oz/¹/₄ cup flour
salt and freshly ground black pepper

Peppercorn sauce
2 x 15ml sp/2 tbs corn or sunflower oil
150ml/¹/₄ pint/²/₃ cup red wine
150ml/¹/₄ pint/²/₃ cup fish stock
1 x 150ml/5fl oz carton/²/₃ cup half-fat crème fraiche
2 tomatoes, chopped
2 x 5ml sp/2 tsp peppercorns, crushed

1   Coat the fish with the flour, to which salt and pepper have been
    added. Heat the oil in a frying pan and cook the fish for about 5 min-
    utes on each side until it is just tender. Remove the fish to a heated
    serving dish and keep it warm.
2   Add the wine to the juices in the pan, scraping the pan to ensure that
    all the sediment is incorporated into the sauce. Boil until the wine has
    reduced to 3 tbs. Add the stock, stir well and boil until it has reduced
    to half the original quantity. Add the crème fraiche and stir over a low
    heat (do not boil or the crème fraiche will curdle) until the sauce is
    smooth. Add the tomatoes and peppercorns and adjust the seasoning
    if necessary. Heat until the sauce is just about to boil, then pour it over
    the fish and serve immediately with vegetables and potatoes.

Summer Fish

▶ **CHO neg** ▶ **CALORIES 1030**   *serves 4*

salt and freshly ground black pepper
4 white fish fillets
4 rashers/4 slices lean streaky bacon
3 courgettes, sliced
pinch dried tarragon
3 x 15ml sp/3 tbs dry vermouth
150ml/5fl oz carton/$^2/_3$ cup half-fat crème fraiche

1 Season the fish with salt and freshly ground black pepper and wrap a bacon rasher around each fillet, then put them in a lightly greased baking dish. Arrange the courgettes around the fish and sprinkle the tarragon over them.
2 Mix the vermouth and crème fraiche together and pour it over the fish.
3 Cover the dish and bake at 350°F/180°F/gas mark 4 for 20 minutes or until the fish is tender.
4 Serve with vegetables and rice.

Steamed Fish and Vegetables

▶ **CHO neg** ▶ **CALORIES 1200** *serves 6*

1 x 15ml sp/1 tbs olive or sunflower oil
1 onion, sliced
4 carrots, cut into julienne strips
3 sticks celery, cut into thin strips
1 bulb fennel, cut into thin strips
150ml/$\frac{1}{4}$ pint/$\frac{2}{3}$ cup dry white wine
150ml/$\frac{1}{4}$ pint/$\frac{2}{3}$ cup fish stock
pinch mixed herbs
salt and freshly ground black pepper
approx. 900g/2 lb halibut on the bone

1 Heat the oil in a shallow pan large enough to accommodate the fish and that has a tight-fitting lid. Add the onion, carrots, celery and fennel and cook for 2–3 minutes. Add the wine and bring it to the boil for 3 minutes to reduce it. Then add the stock, herbs and seasonings. Put the fish on top of the vegetables, cover and steam it over a low heat for about 20 minutes until the fish is cooked.

2 Remove the fish, put the vegetables onto a warmed serving dish and place the fish on top. Pour the sauce over the fish and serve immediately with potatoes.

Salmon Parcels

▶ CHO neg ▶ CALORIES 850 *serves 4*

4 salmon steaks
25g/1oz/2 tbs low-fat spread
4 bay leaves
4 sprigs parsley
1 onion, quartered
4 slices lemon
salt and freshly ground black pepper

1   Put each salmon steak on a square of foil and dot each one with the
    low-fat spread. Top with a bay leaf, a sprig of parsley, quarter of onion,
    slice of lemon and seasonings.
2   Wrap the steaks in the foil and put the parcels in an ovenproof dish.
    Barely cover the bottom of the dish with water and bake at 350°F/
    180°C/gas mark 4 for 15–20 minutes or until the salmon is tender.
    Serve immediately with new potatoes and vegetables.

Fish Cakes

▶ CHO 60g ▶ CALORIES 550　　　　　　　　　　*makes 4*

225g/8oz/1⅓ cups smoked haddock, cooked and flaked
225g/8oz/1 cup potatoes, boiled and mashed
1 x 15ml sp/1 tbs fresh parsley, chopped
1 x 5ml sp/1 tsp lemon juice
salt and freshly ground black pepper
a little olive or sunflower oil for frying

Coating
1 size 3 egg, beaten
50g/2oz/½ cup wholemeal breadcrumbs

1　In a bowl, mix the fish, potatoes, parsley, lemon juice and salt and pepper, binding them together with 1 tbs milk if needed. Shape them into 4 cakes and dip them in the beaten egg, then coat them in the breadcrumbs.
2　Heat the oil (about 3 tbs should be enough) and fry the fish cakes for 5–7 minutes on each side or until they are golden brown then serve with baked beans.

7 vegetarian dishes

Vegetarian meals generally contain more protein and fibre than meat or fish-based meals. They are often more colourful and have a wonderful texture. They are more economical too. Pasta, rice, beans and other pulses are ideal for fast meals as they are quick to prepare and very versatile when combined with different sauces or fillings.

Whether you are vegetarian or not, the recipes in this section are tasty and offer imaginative ways of eating healthily.

Pasta and Pesto Sauce

▶ CHO 150g ▶ CALORIES 2210   *serves 4*

75g/3oz or 5 x 15ml sp/5 tbs fresh basil
50g/2oz/$^1/_3$ cup pine nuts
2–3 cloves garlic, crushed
1 x 1.25ml sp/$^1/_4$ tsp salt
freshly ground black pepper
150ml/$^1/_4$ pint/$^2/_3$ cup olive or rapeseed oil
2 x 15ml sp/2 tbs Parmesan cheese, finely grated
175g–225g/6–8 oz/$^1/_2$ lb wholewheat pasta, cooked

1   Put the basil, pine nuts, garlic and salt in a blender or food processor
    and blend for 1–2 minutes.
2   Slowly add the oil, a little at a time, then stir in the cheese by hand.
3   Toss it well with the freshly cooked *al dente* pasta.

Vegetable Lasagne

▶ **CHO 40g** ▶ **CALORIES 1120**   *serves 4–6*

Filling

1 x 15ml sp/1 tbs olive or sunflower oil
1 onion, sliced
1 clove garlic, crushed
1 green pepper, deseeded and chopped
2 medium carrots, peeled and thinly sliced
100g/4oz/1$\frac{1}{2}$ cups button mushrooms, sliced
1 x 400g/14oz can/1$\frac{3}{4}$ cups tomatoes
1 x 5ml sp/1 tsp mixed herbs
salt and freshly ground black pepper
225g/8oz/1 cup frozen spinach, defrosted and drained
6 slices pre-cooked lasagne

White sauce

15g/$\frac{1}{2}$oz/1 tbs polyunsaturated margarine
15g/$\frac{1}{2}$oz/1 tbs wholemeal flour
150ml/$\frac{1}{4}$ pint/$\frac{2}{3}$ cup skimmed milk
25g/1oz/$\frac{1}{4}$ cup reduced-fat or vegetarian cheddar cheese, grated

Topping

25g/1oz/$\frac{1}{4}$ cup reduced-fat cheddar cheese, grated
25g/1oz/2 tbs unsalted cashew nuts

1   Heat the oil in a pan and lightly sauté the onion and garlic in the oil. Add the pepper, carrot and mushrooms and cook for about 5 minutes. Stir in the tomatoes, herbs and season to taste with salt and freshly ground black pepper. Allow to simmer for 5–10 minutes, stirring occasionally.

2   Meanwhile, make the white sauce. Melt the margarine, stir in the flour and cook for 1 minute. Gradually stir in the milk and bring to the boil, stirring continuously until the sauce has thickened. Stir in the cheese and season to taste.

3   Layer the bolognese mixture, with the spinach and lasagne sheets in alternate layers in an oblong dish, ending with a layer of lasagne. Cover the top with the cheese sauce and sprinkle with the cashew nuts and the remaining cheese. Bake at 350°F/180°C/gas mark 4 for 30–35 minutes.

4   Serve with salad.

Red Lentil Lasagne

▶ CHO 220g ▶ CALORIES 1800

serves 6

225g/8oz/1 cup red lentils
1 x 15ml sp/1 tbs olive or sunflower oil
1 large onion, chopped
2 cloves garlic, crushed
1 green pepper, deseeded and chopped
100g/4oz/1$^{1}/_{2}$ cups mushrooms, sliced
1 x 5ml sp/1 tsp dried basil
1 x 5ml sp/1 tsp dried oregano
1 x 400g/14oz can/1$^{3}/_{4}$ cups chopped tomatoes
1 x 5ml sp/1 tsp yeast extract
275ml/$^{1}/_{2}$ pint/1$^{1}/_{3}$ cups water
1 bay leaf
salt and freshly ground black pepper
8 sheets pre-cooked spinach lasagne (lasagne verde)

White sauce

25g/1oz/2 tbs low-fat spread
25g/1oz/$^{1}/_{4}$ cup wholemeal flour
275ml/$^{1}/_{2}$ pint/1$^{1}/_{3}$ cups skimmed milk
1 x 5ml sp/1 tsp mustard powder
salt and freshly ground black pepper
75g/3oz/$^{3}/_{4}$ cup reduced-fat vegetarian cheese, grated

1   Bring the lentils to the boil in plenty of unsalted water. Boil them fast for 10 minutes, then drain them.

2   Heat the oil in a pan and gently fry the onion and garlic over a moderate heat for 5 minutes. Add the pepper and mushrooms and cook for 5 minutes, stirring from time to time.

3   Add the basil, oregano and drained lentils and cook gently for 2–3 minutes. Stir in the tomatoes and their juice, the yeast extract, water and bay leaf. Bring to the boil, cover and simmer for 15–20 minutes until the lentils are soft. Season with salt and freshly ground black pepper, then remove the bay leaf.

4   Next, make the white sauce. Melt the low-fat spread in a small pan and stir in the flour. Cook it over a gentle heat from 2–3 minutes, stirring. Remove the pan from the heat and gradually stir in the milk. Bring to the boil, stirring all the time, until the sauce thickens. Cook gently for 1–2 minutes. Remove the pan from the heat and beat in the mustard powder and seasoning and a third of the cheese.

5   In a rectangular dish, layer the lentil sauce and lasagne sheets, finishing with a layer of lasagne. Pour the cheese sauce over the top and sprinkle the remaining cheese over it.

6   Bake the lasagne in the oven at 350°F/180°C/gas mark 4 for 30–35 minutes until the cheese has melted, is bubbling and golden brown.

Vegetarian Paella

▶ CHO 40g ▶ CALORIES 630   *serves 2–4*

1 x 15ml sp/1 tbs olive or sunflower oil
2 onions, peeled and chopped
2 cloves of garlic, crushed
100g/4oz/$\frac{1}{2}$ cup brown rice
275ml/$\frac{1}{2}$ pint/1$\frac{1}{3}$ cups vegetable stock
pinch dried basil
2 courgettes, washed and sliced
1 red pepper, deseeded and sliced
1 x 227g/8oz can/1 cup tomatoes
freshly ground black pepper
50g/2oz/$\frac{1}{2}$ cup reduced-fat cheddar cheese, grated
15g/$\frac{1}{2}$oz/2 tbs flaked almonds

1   Heat the oil in a pan and add the onions and garlic. Add the rice and
    cook for a further few minutes coating the grains well with the oil. Add
    the stock and basil, bring to the boil, reduce the heat, cover and
    simmer for 25–30 minutes. Add the courgettes, pepper and tomatoes.
    Season with black pepper and cook for about 10 minutes until the rice
    is cooked and the vegetables are tender.
2   Spoon the mixture into an ovenproof dish. Sprinkle the cheese and
    almonds over the top and grill until lightly browned. Serve immedi-
    ately with salad.

Three-Bean Cassoulet

▶ CHO 80g ▶ CALORIES 770   *serves 4*

1 onion, peeled and sliced
1 clove garlic, crushed
1 x 400g/14oz can/2 cups flageolet beans, drained
1 x 225g/8oz can/1¼ cups red kidney beans, drained and refreshed
    under cold running water
100g/4oz/1 cup cut green beans, cooked
1 x 225g/8oz can/1 cup tomatoes
pinch mixed herbs
salt and freshly ground black pepper
150ml/¼ pint/⅔ cup vegetable stock
25g/1oz/2 tbs sunflower seeds, toasted

1   Put all the ingredients, except the sunflower seeds, into a flameproof
    casserole and bring to the boil. Simmer for about 20 minutes, stirring
    occasionally.
2   Sprinkle the sunflower seeds over the top just before you serve with
    rice or potatoes.

Bean and Vegetable Stew

▶ CHO 100g ▶ CALORIES 1020   *serves 4–6*

1 x 15ml sp/1 tbs corn or sunflower oil
2 cloves garlic, crushed
450g/1 lb leeks, sliced
1 large carrot, sliced
225g/8oz/3 cups mushrooms, sliced
1 x 15ml sp/1 tbs paprika
1 x 15ml sp/1 tbs light soy sauce
275ml/$\frac{1}{2}$ pint/1$\frac{1}{3}$ cups vegetable stock
1 x 225g/8oz can/1$\frac{1}{4}$ cups red kidney beans, drained and refreshed
   under cold running water
salt and freshly ground black pepper

Dumplings
100g/4oz/1 cup self-raising 100 per cent wholemeal flour
50g/2oz/$\frac{1}{4}$ cup vegetable suet
pinch salt
1 x 15ml sp/1 tbs parsley, chopped
a little water to bind

1   Heat the oil in a flameproof casserole. Add the garlic, leeks, carrot and mushrooms and sauté them until they are tender. Add the paprika, soy sauce and stock and bring to the boil. Add the kidney beans, salt and freshly ground black pepper and simmer for 20 minutes.

2   Meanwhile, make the dumplings. Mix all the ingredients together to make a firm dough. Shape it into 6–8 dumplings and arrange them on top of the stew. Cover the casserole and simmer gently for 20 minutes until the dumplings are light and fluffy, then serve straight away with potatoes.

Chickpea Moussaka

▶ CHO 160g ▶ CALORIES 1270   *serves 4*

1 large aubergine
350g/12oz/³⁄₄ lb potatoes, peeled
1 onion, peeled and finely chopped
2 cloves garlic, crushed
1 x 15ml sp/1 tbs olive or sunflower oil
50g/2oz/³⁄₄ cup mushrooms, sliced
1 x 400g/14oz can/1³⁄₄ cup chopped tomatoes
2 x 5ml sp/2 tsp dried oregano
1 x 15ml sp/1 tbs Worcestershire sauce
dash of Tabasco sauce
1 x 400g/14oz can/2¹⁄₄ cups chickpeas, drained
sea salt and freshly ground black pepper

Topping

2 size 3 eggs, beaten
1 x 5ml sp/1 tsp cumin seeds, toasted (optional)
1 x 150ml/5 fl oz carton/²⁄₃ cup low-fat natural yogurt
tomato slices and parsley, to garnish

1   Prick and trim the aubergines and bake them in a 350°F/180°C/gas
    mark 4 oven for 20–30 minutes, then slice (leaving the oven on).
2   Boil the potatoes until they are tender, then slice them thickly.
3   Gently fry the onion and garlic in the oil for 4–5 minutes. Add the
    mushrooms, tomatoes, oregano, Worcestershire and Tabasco sauces,
    chickpeas and season with salt and freshly ground black pepper. Cook
    gently for 10 minutes, adjusting the seasoning if necessary.

4   Arrange layers of aubergine, potato and vegetable sauce in an oven-proof casserole dish, finishing with a layer of aubergine. Beat together the topping ingredients and spoon the mixture over the moussaka. Bake in the oven for 25–30 minutes.

Mixed Bean Hot Pot

▶ CHO 120g ▶ CALORIES 660   *serves 3–4*

1 x 225g/8oz/1¼ cups tin cannellini beans, drained and rinsed
100g/4oz/1 cup French beans
1 x 227g/8oz can/1 cup tomatoes
1 x 15ml sp/1 tbs tomato purée
1 clove garlic, crushed
1 x 5ml sp/1 tsp mixed herbs
salt and freshly ground black pepper
225g/8oz/2¾ cups potatoes, parboiled and sliced
25g/1oz/¼ cup reduced-fat vegetarian cheddar cheese, grated

1   Mix all the ingredients together, except the potatoes and cheese, and
    pour into an ovenproof dish. Arrange the sliced potatoes on top of the
    mixture and sprinkle the cheese over them.
2   Cook at 325°F/170°C/gas mark 3 for 45 minutes–1 hour or until the
    potatoes are cooked.

Braised Green Lentils

▶ CHO 110g ▶ CALORIES 990   *serves 4*

225g/8oz/1 cup green lentils
1 x 15ml sp/1 tbs olive or sunflower oil
1 onion, peeled and finely chopped
1 small potato, cut into small pieces
1 carrot, scrubbed and diced
1 leek, washed and finely sliced
2 tomatoes, seeded and diced
275ml/$\frac{1}{2}$ pint/1$\frac{1}{3}$ cups vegetable stock
1 small garlic clove, crushed
salt and freshly ground black pepper
1 x 5ml sp/1 tsp white wine vinegar

1   Wash the lentils thoroughly and leave to drain.
2   Heat the oil in a pan and sauté the remaining vegetables gently, stir-
    ring all the time, for about 3–4 minutes. Add the stock, garlic and
    drained lentils and bring to the boil. Simmer until the lentils are just
    tender (about 7–10 minutes).
3   Season to taste with salt and freshly ground black pepper and add the
    vinegar.

▶ **Note to Cooks** *This mixture can be used to make a vegetarian Shepherd's Pie by piping creamed potato over the top.*

Lentil Moussaka

▶ CHO 150g ▶ CALORIES 1310   *serves 6*

2 medium aubergines, sliced
2 x 15ml sp/2 tbs olive oil
2 medium onions, peeled and chopped
100g/4oz/½ cup green lentils, cooked
1 x 5ml sp/1 tsp mixed herbs
1 x 5ml sp/1 tsp nutmeg, grated
1 x 15ml sp/1 tbs tomato purée
1 x 400g/14oz can/1¾ cups tomatoes, drained and chopped,
    reserving the juice
600g/22oz/3 cups potatoes, parboiled and sliced

White sauce
25g/1oz/2 tbs low-fat spread
25g/1oz/¼ cup flour
275ml/½ pint/1⅓ cups skimmed milk
1 size 3 egg
salt and freshly ground black pepper
1 x 2.5ml sp/½ tsp nutmeg, grated
1 tomato, sliced

1   Sprinkle the aubergine slices with salt and leave to stand for 30 min-
    utes to remove the bitter juices. Pat dry with kitchen paper towels.
    Then heat the oil in a pan and fry the aubergines until they are golden
    brown. Set aside.
2   Fry the onions in the pan until they are soft, then add the lentils, herbs,
    nutmeg, tomato purée and tomato juice. Simmer for 5 minutes.

3   Assemble the moussaka by arranging a layer of aubergine slices in an ovenproof dish, followed by slices of potato, chopped tomatoes and the lentil mixture. Repeat until all ingredients are used, ending with a layer of aubergine slices.

4   To make the sauce, melt the low-fat spread in a pan, stir in the flour, then gradually add the milk. Bring to the boil, stirring all the time, then reduce the heat and simmer for 2–3 minutes until the sauce is thickened, stirring continuously. Remove the pan from the heat, season to taste and allow to cool slightly before beating in the egg quickly until the sauce is glossy. Pour the sauce over the moussaka. Garnish with the sliced tomato. Bake at 375°F/190°C/gas mark 5 for 45 minutes and serve hot.

Mung Bean and Vegetable Cottage Pie

▶ CHO 190g ▶ CALORIES 1220   *serves 4–6*

2 x 5ml sp/2 tsp sunflower oil
1 onion, finely chopped
2 carrots, finely chopped
3 sticks celery, diced
225g/8oz/1¼ cups mung beans, cooked
2 x 5ml sp/2 tsp cayenne pepper
1 x 5ml sp/1 tsp fresh marjoram, chopped
1 x 5ml sp/1 tsp fresh sage, chopped
1 x 15ml sp/1 tbs tomato purée
1 x 5ml sp/1 tsp yeast extract
275ml/½ pint/1⅓ cups vegetable stock
salt and freshly ground black pepper
450g/1 lb/2⅔ cups potatoes, peeled and diced
4 x 15ml sp/4 tbs skimmed milk
15g/½ oz/1 tbs sunflower seeds

1   Preheat the oven to 350°F/180°C/gas mark 4.
2   Heat the oil in a large pan and fry the onion, carrots and celery for 5 minutes. Add the cooked mung beans, cayenne pepper, herbs, tomato purée, yeast extract and stock. Cover and simmer gently for 10–15 minutes. Season to taste with salt and freshly ground black pepper.
3   Meanwhile, boil the potatoes until they are cooked. Drain and mash them with the milk. Put the bean mixture into a large casserole dish and top this with the mashed potato. Sprinkle the sunflower seeds over the top and bake in the preheated oven for 30–40 minutes, until the top is golden brown.

Courgette and Sweetcorn Gratin

▶ CHO 110g ▶ CALORIES 1100   *serves 4–6*

100g/4oz/¹⁄₂ cup red lentils
2 x 5ml sp/2 tsp olive or sunflower oil
1 onion, peeled and finely chopped
1 clove garlic, crushed
1 x 15ml sp/1 tbs tomato purée
50g/2oz/¹⁄₂ cup oatmeal
1 x 15ml sp/1 tbs lemon juice
1 x 5ml sp/1 tsp dried mixed herbs
salt and freshly ground black pepper

Filling

100g/4oz/1 cup courgettes, finely diced
100g/4oz/1 cup red pepper, deseeded and finely diced
1 size 3 egg, beaten
1 x 15ml sp/1 tbs wholemeal flour
100ml/4fl oz/¹⁄₃ cup skimmed milk
100g/4oz/²⁄₃ cup canned sweetcorn
salt and freshly ground black pepper
50g/2oz/¹⁄₂ cup vegetarian cheese, grated

1   Boil the lentils in plenty of unsalted water. Boil them fast for 10 minutes then drain them well.

2   Heat the oil in a pan and gently fry the onion for 2–3 minutes. Add the garlic and fry it for 1 minute. Remove the pan from the heat and mix in the lentils, tomato purée, oatmeal, lemon juice and herbs. Season to taste with salt and freshly ground black pepper. The mixture should be

thick enough to hold together, but if the lentils are still a little wet, return the pan to the heat to dry it out a little, stirring, or add a little more oatmeal. Press the mixture around the sides and bottom of a 20cm/8 inch flan dish.

3   For the filling, lightly steam the courgettes and pepper for 4 minutes or until tender. Blend the egg with the flour, then add the milk. Stir in the cooked courgettes and sweetcorn and season well. Spoon the filling into the flan dish, cover the top with the cheese. Bake at 375°F/190°C/gas mark 5 for 30–35 minutes, or until the filling has set and serve hot with jacket potatoes and salad.

Stir-Fried Vegetables

▶ CHO neg ▶ CALORIES 400   *serves 4*

1 x 15ml sp/1 tbs olive or sunflower oil
4 carrots, cut into strips
½ cauliflower, broken into florets
175g/6oz/1 cup baby sweetcorn
100g/4oz/1 cup runner beans, cut into pieces
100g/4oz/1½ cups button mushrooms, sliced
225g/8oz/4 cups beansprouts
2 x 5ml sp/2 tsp soy sauce

1   Heat the oil in a wok or large frying pan.
2   Add the carrots, cauliflower, sweetcorn and beans and stir for 1–2
    minutes. Add the remaining vegetables and cook 1–2 more minutes.
    Toss the vegetables in the soy sauce and serve immediately with rice.

Vegetable Casserole

▶ CHO 10g ▶ CALORIES 190   *serves 4*

1 small swede (about 225g/8oz), peeled and finely diced
2 carrots, peeled and sliced
1 large onion, peeled and chopped
4 sticks celery, chopped
1 x 400g/14oz can/1¾ cups tomatoes
salt and freshly ground black pepper
pinch ground nutmeg
about 150ml/¼ pint/⅔ cup vegetable stock

1   Mix the prepared vegetables together in a 1.75ltr/3 pint casserole
    dish. Season to taste with salt and freshly ground black pepper.
2   Pour the tomatoes and some of the stock over the vegetables and
    cook at 350°F/180°C/gas mark 4 for 1–1¼ hours, or until the vege-
    tables are tender. Add some extra stock if the mixture begins to get
    a little dry.
3   Serve with jacket potatoes.

Cheesy Leek and Potato Casserole

▶ CHO 110g ▶ CALORIES 930   *serves 4–6*

450g/1 lb leeks, sliced
1 onion, peeled and finely sliced
450g/1 lb potatoes, thickly sliced
25g/1oz/2 tbs low-fat spread
25g/1oz/¼ cup wholemeal flour
275ml/½ pint/1⅓ cups skimmed milk
1 x 2.5ml sp/½ tsp mustard
sea salt
1 x 2.5ml sp/½ tsp paprika
1 x 2.5ml sp/½ tsp ground cumin
50g/2oz/½ cup vegetarian cheese, grated
1 x 2.5ml sp/½ tsp cumin seeds (optional)

1   Preheat the oven to 350°F/180°C/gas mark 4.
2   Steam the leeks over a large pan of simmering water for 8 minutes.
3   Meanwhile, cover the potato slices with water, bring to the boil and
    simmer gently for 8 minutes. Drain well.
4   While the potatoes are cooking, melt the low-fat spread in a pan, add
    the flour and cook gently, stirring, for 2–3 minutes. Remove the pan
    from the heat and gradually stir in the milk. Return the pan to the heat,
    bring the sauce to the boil, stirring constantly, and cook gently for 2–3
    minutes. Stir in the mustard, seasoning and spices.
5   Layer the leek, onion and potato slices in a casserole or ovenproof dish.
    Pour the sauce over them and top with the grated cheese. Sprinkle the
    cumin seeds over, if using. Bake in the preheated oven for 30 minutes,
    or until the top is golden brown and the vegetables are cooked.

Mixed Vegetable Curry

▶ CHO 50g ▶ CALORIES 470   *serves 4–6*

2 x 5ml sp/2 tsp olive or sunflower oil
1 x 5ml sp/1 tsp cumin seeds
1 x 5ml sp/1 tsp coriander seeds
1 large onion, peeled and finely chopped
3 cloves garlic, crushed
1 x 5ml sp/1 tsp garam masala
1 x 2.5ml sp/$^1/_2$ tsp chilli powder
2 medium potatoes, finely diced
100g/4oz/1 cup cauliflower, cut into florets
2 courgettes, sliced
1 leek, sliced
1 green pepper, deseeded and cut into strips
25g/1oz/$^1/_4$ cup wholemeal flour
1 x 400g/14oz can/1$^3/_4$ cups chopped tomatoes
150ml/1/4 pint/$^2/_3$ cup vegetable stock
2 x 15ml sp/2 tbs low-fat natural yogurt
salt and freshly ground black pepper

1   Heat the oil in a large pan and gently cook the cumin and coriander
    seeds for 3–4 minutes until the seeds are turning brown.
2   Add the onion, garlic, garam masala and chilli powder and cook gently
    for 2 minutes.
3   Add the potato, cauliflower, courgette, leek and green pepper and
    continue cooking for 3 minutes, stirring well to ensure that the vegeta-
    bles are well coated in spices. Sprinkle the flour over them and cook
    for 1 minute.

4   Add the tomatoes and their juice together with the stock.

5   Bring to the boil, cover and simmer gently for 40–45 minutes, stirring occasionally, adding a little extra stock if the sauce thickens a little too much.

6   When the vegetables are tender, add the yogurt. Adjust the seasoning to taste and serve hot with rice.

▶ *Notes to Cooks The flavours of the curry will have more time to develop if the dish is made a day in advance. 1–2 tablespoons of curry powder may be used in place of the various spices if you do not have them.*

Stir-Fried Vegetable Salad

▶ CHO neg ▶ CALORIES 335   *serves 3*

1 x 15ml sp/1 tbs olive oil or sunflower oil
1 clove garlic, crushed
1 small piece root ginger, peeled and crushed
1 x 2.5ml sp/$\frac{1}{2}$ tsp coriander seed, crushed
1 medium onion, peeled and chopped
100g/4oz/1 cup baby sweetcorn, trimmed
3 small courgettes, cut into wedges
1 small red pepper, deseeded and sliced
1 small green pepper, deseeded and sliced
salt and freshly ground black pepper
1 x 15ml sp/1 tbs light soy sauce
1 x 5ml sp/1 tsp fresh coriander leaves to garnish

1   Heat the oil in a wok or large frying pan with a close-fitting lid.
2   Add the garlic, ginger and coriander seed and cook for a minute. Add
    the onion, sweetcorn and courgettes. Cover and cook for a few
    minutes.
3   Add the peppers, cover and cook for 5 minutes, stirring occasionally.
    Season with salt and freshly ground black pepper.
4   Remove the pan from the heat and add the soy sauce. Serve warm,
    garnished with the fresh coriander leaves, accompanied by rice.

Savoury Crumble

▶ CHO 180g ▶ CALORIES 1500   *serves 4–6*

2 x 5ml sp/2 tsp olive or sunflower oil
1 onion, peeled and chopped
100g/4oz/1$\frac{1}{2}$ cups mushrooms, sliced
100g/4oz/$\frac{2}{3}$ cup carrots, sliced
1 small cauliflower, cut into florets
2 x 5ml sp/2 tsp fresh rosemary, chopped
1 x 15ml sp/1 tbs wholemeal flour
275ml/$\frac{1}{2}$ pint/1$\frac{1}{3}$ cups vegetable stock
salt and freshly ground black pepper
1 x 425g/15oz can/2$\frac{1}{3}$ cups butter beans, drained
1 x 225g/8oz can/1$\frac{1}{4}$ cups kidney beans, drained and refreshed under
    cold running water

Topping
50g/2oz/$\frac{1}{2}$ cup porridge or jumbo oats
50g/2oz/$\frac{1}{2}$ cup 100 per cent wholemeal flour
25g/1oz/3 tbs hazelnuts, chopped
25g/1oz/2 tbs low-fat spread

1   Heat the oil in a large frying pan with a close-fitting lid over a moder-
    ate heat and fry the onion, mushrooms, carrots and cauliflower. Cover
    and cook for 5 minutes, stirring frequently. Then, sprinkle the rosemary
    and flour over the vegetables and cook for 2–3 minutes.
2   Pour on the stock, bring to the boil and simmer gently for 2 minutes.
    Add salt and freshly ground black pepper to taste, then the butter and
    kidney beans. Pour the mixture into a casserole or ovenproof dish.

3   For the topping, mix together the oats, flour, hazelnuts and low-fat spread. Sprinkle it on top of the vegetables and bake at 350°F/180°C/gas mark 4 for 30 minutes. Serve hot.

Stuffed Pepper

▶ CHO 30g ▶ CALORIES 210   *serves 1*

1 medium green or red pepper
1 x 5ml sp/1 tsp corn or sunflower oil
25g/1oz/1 tbs brown rice, cooked
25g/1oz/2 tbs frozen peas
25g/1oz/2 tbs frozen sweetcorn
1 x 15ml sp/1 tbs raisins
salt and freshly ground black pepper

1   Slice the top off the pepper and remove the seeds and any white pith.
2   Put the pepper in a saucepan of water and bring to the boil. Simmer for 10 minutes or until it is tender. Drain and keep it warm.
3   Heat the oil in a saucepan, add the rice, vegetables and raisins and season to taste with salt and freshly ground black pepper. Heat thoroughly, spoon the mixture into the pepper and serve.

Nut Roast

▶ CHO 60g ▶ CALORIES 1220   *makes 6 slices*

1 onion, peeled and finely chopped
25g/1oz/2 tbs low-fat spread
225g/8oz/1^2/$_3$ cups mixed nuts, chopped
100g/4oz/2 cups wholemeal breadcrumbs
275ml/^{1}/$_2$ pint/1^1/$_3$ cups vegetable stock
2 x 5ml sp/2 tsp yeast extract
pinch mixed herbs
salt and freshly ground black pepper
slices of tomato to garnish

1   Sauté the onions until transparent in the low-fat spread that you have melted in a pan.

2   In a large bowl, combine all the other ingredients (reserving 1 tbs of the breadcrumbs) and mix together well. The mixture should be loose.

3   Turn the mixture into a lightly greased 450g/1 lb loaf tin and sprinkle the reserved breadcrumbs over the top. Bake the loaf at 350°F/180°C/gas mark 4 for 30 minutes or until it is golden brown. Allow it to cool before you turn it out, then garnish it with the sliced tomatoes.

Basic Pancake Mixture

▶ **CHO 130g** ▶ **CALORIES 800**   *makes 12*

150g/5oz/1¼ cups plain flour
pinch salt
2 size 3 eggs, lightly beaten
275ml/½ pint/1⅓ cups skimmed milk
150ml/¼ pint/⅔ cup water
1 x 5ml sp/1 tsp corn or sunflower oil

1   Sift the flour into a bowl and add a pinch of salt. Make a well in the
    centre and pour in the eggs.
2   Gradually add the milk and water to the well, stirring round the edge
    of the well until all the flour becomes amalgamated and smooth. Then
    mix in the oil and leave to stand for 2–3 hours.
3   When the batter has stood for this time, lightly grease and heat a
    heavy-bottomed frying pan. Cook approximately 1 tbs of the mixture
    at a time, spreading it over the pan. Loosen the edges of the pancakes
    from the pan before tossing. Allow them to cook for 1 minute on each
    side.

Fillings

▶ CHO neg ▶ CALORIES 280

Ratatouille Filling

1 x 400g/14oz can/1¾ cups chopped tomatoes
2 onions, peeled and chopped
1 small courgette, sliced
1 green pepper, deseeded and sliced
1–2 cloves garlic, crushed
pinch mixed herbs
salt and freshly ground black pepper
50g/2oz/½ cup reduced-fat cheddar cheese, grated

1   Put all the ingredients except the cheese in a saucepan and simmer for 10–15 minutes, seasoning to taste with salt and freshly ground black pepper.
2   Fill the pancakes with the ratatouille – putting 2–3 tbs of it in the middle of each pancake – then roll them up and put them in an oven-proof dish. Sprinkle the cheese over them and bake for 10 minutes at 350°F/ 180°C/gas mark 4.

▶ CHO 30g ▶ CALORIES 540

Sweetcorn and Mushroom Filling

25g/1oz/2 tbs low-fat spread
225g/8oz/3 cups mushrooms, sliced
1 x 300g/11oz can/1½ cups sweetcorn, drained

Cheese sauce

25g/1oz/2 tbs low-fat spread
25g/1oz/¼ cup flour
275ml/½ pint/1⅓ cups skimmed milk
salt and freshly ground black pepper
25g/1oz/¼ cup reduced-fat cheddar cheese, grated
salt and freshly ground black pepper

1   Melt the low-fat spread in a pan, lightly sauté the mushrooms.
2   Meanwhile, make the cheese sauce. Melt the low-fat spread in a pan,
    stir in the flour and cook for 1 minute. Then lower the heat and gradu-
    ally add the milk, stirring all the time. Bring the sauce to a boil and stir
    quickly until the sauce thickens. Add the cheese and stir until it has
    melted, then add the mushrooms and sweetcorn. Season to taste with
    salt and freshly ground black pepper.
3   Use to fill the pancakes in the same way as for the Ratatouille filling.

8 salads and side dishes

Accompaniments to the main course provide colour, texture and a tasty diversion. By using low-fat, high-fibre ingredients, the selection of appetizing recipes in this section gives you all of these and more – health-promoting delicious morsels. Try them on their own, too, for lunches or snacks.

Wholewheat Pasta Salad

▶ CHO 40g ▶ CALORIES 440   *serves 2*

50g/2oz/1 cup wholewheat pasta, cooked
1 medium or 2 small carrots, sliced
$\frac{1}{2}$ green pepper, deseeded and cut into strips
2 stalks celery, chopped
1 x 2.5ml sp/$\frac{1}{2}$ tsp garlic powder
1 x 15ml sp/1 tbs Worcestershire or soy sauce
fresh parsley, chopped, to garnish

1   Mix all the ingredients, except the parsley, together in a bowl.
2   Garnish the salad with the chopped parsley.

Waldorf Salad

▶ CHO 60g ▶ CALORIES 570   *serves 4–6*

3 red apples, diced
2 x 15ml sp/2 tbs lemon juice
50g/2oz/$\frac{1}{2}$ cup walnuts, chopped
1 head celery, chopped
300g/10fl oz carton/1$\frac{1}{3}$ cups low-fat natural yogurt
a few lettuce leaves to garnish

1   Put all but a third of the apple in a bowl and drizzle the lemon juice
    over to prevent it browning. Mix the nuts, celery and natural yogurt
    with the apple.
2   Arrange the lettuce leaves and salad on a serving dish. Use the
    reserved apple to garnish the salad.

Italian Bean Salad

▶ CHO 50g ▶ CALORIES 670   *serves 4*

1 x 425g/15oz can/2$^{1}/_{3}$ cups cannellini beans, drained
1 x 200g/7oz can/1 cup tuna in brine, drained
1 small onion, peeled and sliced
4 x 15ml sp/4 tbs Mustard Dressing recipe (see page 141)

1   Put all the ingredients into a bowl and toss together until they are well
    mixed.
2   Chill in the refrigerator before serving.

Red Kidney Beans with Walnuts

▶ CHO 30g ▶ CALORIES 800 *serves 4*

1 x 227g/8oz can/1¼ cups red kidney beans, drained and refreshed
   under cold running water
1 small fennel bulb, finely chopped
1 onion, peeled and sliced
50g/2oz/½ cup walnuts, chopped
3 x 15ml sp/3 tbs olive oil
2–3 x 15ml sp/2–3 tbs fresh parsley, chopped
2 cloves garlic, crushed
salt and freshly ground black pepper

1   Mix the kidney beans, fennel, onion and walnuts together in a salad
    bowl.
2   Season the olive oil with the parsley, garlic and salt and freshly ground
    black pepper. Dress the vegetable mixture with it and leave to mari-
    nate for an hour or so before serving.

Autumn Salad

▶ CHO 40g ▶ CALORIES 680   *serves 6*

1 crispy lettuce, shredded
1 green pepper, deseeded and sliced
2 courgettes, thinly sliced
75g/3oz/^{1}/$_2$ cup green lentils, cooked
1 x Low-calorie French Dressing recipe (see page 140)
salt and freshly ground black pepper
1 x 5ml sp/1 tsp ground cumin
50g/2oz/^{1}/$_2$ cup unsalted peanuts, chopped and toasted

1   Put the lettuce and green pepper into a salad bowl. Add the cour-
    gettes and lentils.
2   Pour the Low-calorie French Dressing over the salad and mix so it
    coats all the ingredients well. Season to taste with salt and freshly
    ground black pepper.
3   Just before serving, toss in the chopped peanuts.

Rice Salad

▶ CHO 145g ▶ CALORIES 1095   *serves 6*

175g/6oz/1 cup brown rice, cooked
225g/8oz/1 cup tomatoes chopped
1 green pepper, deseeded and sliced
10 green olives, stoned and halved
50g/2oz/^{1}/$_2$ cup unsalted peanuts, chopped and toasted
1 x Low-calorie French Dressing recipe (see page 140)
salt and freshly ground black pepper

1   Put the rice into a bowl. Add the tomatoes, pepper, olives and peanuts
     and mix everything together well.
2   Pour in the Low-calorie French Dressing and season to taste with salt
     and freshly ground black pepper.
3   Chill until you are ready to serve.

Rice and Millet Salad

▶ CHO 160g ▶ CALORIES 880   *serves 6–8*

100g/4oz/$\frac{1}{2}$ cup long-grained brown rice
100g/4oz/$\frac{1}{2}$ cup millet
1 onion, finely chopped
6 cardamom pods, slightly crushed
20 coriander seeds, crushed
pinch cinnamon
425ml/$\frac{3}{4}$ pint/2 cups vegetable stock
2 sprigs fresh thyme
salt and freshly ground black pepper
4 stalks celery, trimmed and cut into small chunks
1 red pepper, deseeded and diced
25g/1oz/$\frac{1}{4}$ cup hazelnuts or walnuts, lightly toasted
1 x 15ml sp/1 tbs fresh coriander, roughly chopped

Dressing
1 x 5ml sp/1 tsp light soy sauce
2 x 15ml sp/2 tbs lemon juice

1   Wash the rice and millet and leave them to drain.
2   Meanwhile, sweat the onion and spices over gentle heat in a non-stick
     pan for 2–3 minutes. Add the rice and millet, stirring with a wooden
     spoon, then add the stock and thyme. Stir again to ensure that no
     grains have stuck to the bottom of the pan and season with salt and
     freshly ground black pepper. Bring to the boil, cover and simmer for
     about 20–25 minutes. The grains should now be tender and all the
     liquid should have been absorbed.

3 Tip the rice and millet into a warmed serving bowl and use a fork to separate the grains, removing the thyme and cardamom pods as you go. Leave it to cool before adding the celery, pepper, nuts and coriander. Mix the dressing and pour it over the salad. Mix everything together well and serve.

Prawn and Rice Salad

▶ **CHO 140g** ▶ **CALORIES 1210**   *serves 4–6*

175g/6oz/1 cup brown rice, cooked
225g/8oz/2 cups frozen prawns, defrosted
4 spring onions, finely chopped
1 green pepper, deseeded and chopped
2 tomatoes, chopped
salt and freshly ground black pepper
fresh parsley, chopped, to garnish

Dressing
3 x 15ml sp/3 tbs olive oil
1 x 15ml sp/1 tbs lemon juice
pinch mixed herbs

1   Put the rice in a bowl.
2   Mix the dressing ingredients in a screw-top jar and pour it over the
     rice.
3   Add the prawns, spring onions, peppers, tomatoes and seasoning and
     mix them together well. Serve garnished with the parsley.

Fish Salad Platter

▶ CHO neg ▶ CALORIES 610

serves 4

225g/8oz/1¹⁄₃ cups cod fillet, cooked and flaked
2 x 15ml sp/2 tbs low-calorie French dressing
2 x 5ml sp/2 tsp lemon juice
1 x 200g/7oz can/1 cup tuna in brine, drained
2 size 3 eggs, hard-boiled and quartered
salt and freshly ground black pepper
1 lettuce, washed
3 tomatoes, sliced
1 green pepper, deseeded and sliced
6 black olives, halved, to garnish

1   Put the cod in a bowl. Add the French dressing and lemon juice. Add the tuna and eggs. Toss lightly together and season to taste with salt and freshly ground black pepper.

2   Arrange the lettuce leaves on a platter. Pile the fish mixture on top and arrange the tomato slices and pepper rings around it. Serve garnished with the olives.

Fruit and Vegetable Mixed Salad

▶ CHO 90g ▶ CALORIES 550   *serves 6–8*

3 carrots, peeled and coarsely grated

2 apples, cored and sliced

2 pears, cored and sliced

6 sticks celery, finely sliced

$^1\!/_2$ cucumber, diced

50g/2oz/$^1\!/_3$ cup raisins

1 x 5ml sp/1 tsp lemon juice

salt and freshly ground black pepper

1 x 150g/5fl oz carton/$^2\!/_3$ cup low-fat natural yogurt

1   Put all the prepared fruit and vegetables into a bowl.

2   Add the lemon juice and seasonings to the yogurt.

3   Mix the yogurt dressing with the salad ingredients and chill well before
    serving.

Slimmer's Salad

▶ CHO 10g ▶ CALORIES 640   *serves 4–6*

450g/1 lb/2 cups cottage cheese
1 x 150g/1 x 5fl oz carton/²/₃ cup low-fat natural yogurt
2 x 15ml sp/2 tbs fresh chives, chopped
¹/₂ cucumber, diced
1 red pepper, deseeded and diced
¹/₂ onion, grated
salt and freshly ground black pepper
a few lettuce leaves, shredded, to garnish

1   Combine the cottage cheese with the yogurt, chives, cucumber, and
    pepper.
2   Season to taste with the onion, salt and pepper and toss together well.
3   Serve on a bed of the lettuce.

Low-Calorie French Dressing

▶ CHO neg ▶ CALORIES 100   *makes 100ml/4fl oz*

6 x 15ml sp/6 tbs cider or wine vinegar
1 x 15ml sp/1 tbs olive oil
1 x 2.5ml sp/¹/₂ tsp dry mustard
salt and freshly ground black pepper

1   Measure all the ingredients into a jar with a screw-top lid. Shake them
    together well and store in the refrigerator until the dressing is needed.
2   Shake the jar vigorously before using as the ingredients settle.

▶ *Note to Cooks This recipe will keep for 2–3 days in the refrigerator.*

Mustard Dressing

▶ CHO neg ▶ CALORIES 330   *makes 100ml/4fl oz*

3 x 15ml sp/3 tbs olive oil
2 x 15ml sp/2 tbs cider vinegar
1 x 5ml sp/1 tsp wholegrain mustard
1 small onion, peeled and grated
1 clove garlic, crushed
pinch intense sweetener
salt and freshly ground black pepper

1   Measure all the ingredients into a screw-top jar and shake it until well mixed. Chill the dressing in the refrigerator until you need it.
2   Shake the jar well before serving to remix the ingredients as they tend to settle after the initial making.

▶ *Note to Cooks This recipe will keep for 2–3 days in the refrigerator.*

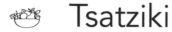 # Tsatziki

▶ CHO 20g ▶ CALORIES 160   *serves 4–6*

2 x 150g/5fl oz cartons/²⁄₃ cup low-fat natural yogurt
10cm/4 inch piece cucumber, diced
1 x 15ml sp/1 tbs fresh mint, chopped
1 clove garlic, crushed (optional)
1 sprig fresh mint to garnish

1   Mix all the ingredients together and chill it well before you serve it.
2   Garnish the Tzatziki with the sprig of mint.

Potato and Sprout Bake

▶ CHO 80g ▶ CALORIES 550   *serves 4–6*

450g/1 lb/2²⁄₃ cups potatoes, peeled and diced
225g/8oz/2 cups Brussels sprouts, peeled and trimmed
15g/¹⁄₂ oz/1 tbs low-fat spread
freshly grated nutmeg
salt and freshly ground black pepper
25g/1oz/¹⁄₄ cup reduced-fat cheddar cheese, grated

1   Cook the potatoes and sprouts in boiling water for about 15 minutes. Drain, then mash them together with the low-fat spread, nutmeg and season with salt and freshly ground black pepper.

2   Spoon the mixture into a heatproof dish, sprinkle the cheese over the top and grill until the cheese is bubbling and golden brown. Serve immediately.

Cooked Chicory

▶ **CHO neg** ▶ **CALORIES 240**   *serves 4*

50g/2oz/¼ cup low-fat spread
450g/1 lb chicory, leaves separated from the stem
pinch salt
pinch intense sweetener
1 lemon, juice of

1   Melt the low-fat spread in a pan and toss the chicory leaves in it. Add
    the salt, sweetener and lemon juice and cover.
2   Cook over a gentle heat for 10 minutes, then serve immediately.

Braised Celery

▶ CHO neg ▶ CALORIES 210 *serves 4*

1 onion, peeled and chopped
1 medium carrot, peeled and chopped
1 clove garlic, crushed
25g/1oz/2 tbs low-fat spread
2 small heads of celery, split into individual sticks
150ml/¼ pint/⅔ cup vegetable stock
salt and freshly ground black pepper
1–2 x 15ml sp/1–2 tbs fresh parsley, chopped

1   Lightly sauté the onion, carrot and garlic in the low-fat spread in a pan
    for 5 minutes. Transfer the vegetables to an ovenproof casserole. Put
    the celery on top of the vegetables. Pour the stock over it and season
    well with salt and freshly ground black pepper.
2   Cover and bake at 350°F/180°C/gas mark 4 for approximately 1–1½
    hours, turning the celery occasionally in the juices.
3   Serve this dish hot, with the parsley sprinkled over it just before
    serving.

Spring Cabbage

▶ CHO neg ▶ CALORIES 360   *serves 4*

25g/1oz/2 tbs low-fat spread
675g/1¹/₂ lb spring cabbage, shredded
1 onion, peeled and chopped
2 rashers/2 slices streaky bacon, rind removed and chopped
pinch grated nutmeg

1   Heat the low-fat spread in a large saucepan, add all the ingredients,
     cover and cook very gently for 20–30 minutes, until the cabbage is just
     tender, stirring frequently.
2   Serve immediately.

Stuffed Mushrooms

▶ CHO 30g ▶ CALORIES 400   *serves 4*

4 large field mushrooms
50g/2oz/1 cup wholemeal breadcrumbs
50g/2oz/$\frac{1}{2}$ cup reduced-fat cheddar cheese, grated
25g/1oz/3 tbs walnuts, finely chopped
pinch mixed herbs
freshly ground black pepper
1 x 15ml sp/1 tbs tomato ketchup

1   Remove the mushroom stalks and chop them finely. Mix them together
    with the remaining ingredients. Spoon equal amounts into each of the
    mushroom caps and put them on a baking sheet.
2   Bake them at 375°F/190°C/gas mark 5 for 10 minutes. Serve as soon
    as they are done.

Peppers à la Provence

▶ CHO neg ▶ CALORIES 260   *serves 4*

1 x 15ml sp/1 tbs olive or sunflower oil
2 medium onions, peeled and sliced
1 clove garlic, crushed
4 peppers (assorted colours), deseeded and sliced
1 x 400g/14oz can/1¾ cups tomatoes
1 x 5ml sp/1 tsp *herbs de Provence*
salt and freshly ground black pepper

1   Heat the oil in a large pan, add the onions and garlic and fry them until
    they are soft. Add the peppers and cook for 5–10 minutes.
2   Stir in the tomatoes, herbs and season to taste with salt and freshly
    ground black pepper. Bring to the boil, then simmer for 15–20
    minutes.
3   Serve either hot or cold.

Sautéed Okra

▶ CHO neg ▶ CALORIES 180   *serves 4*

1 x 15ml sp/1 tbs olive or sunflower oil
1 onion, peeled and chopped
1 x 2.5ml sp/½ tsp chilli powder
1 x 5ml sp/1 tsp ground coriander
1 x 5ml sp/1 tsp garam masala
225g/8oz/½ lb okra
1–2 x 15ml sp/1–2 tbs lemon juice
pinch salt

1   Heat the oil in a pan and fry the onion, chilli powder, coriander and garam masala. Add the okra and lemon juice and a pinch of salt and cook for approximately 5 minutes.
2   Serve immediately.

Stuffed Aubergines

▶ CHO 20g ▶ CALORIES 865　　　　　　　　　　*serves 6*

3 medium aubergines
1 x 15ml sp/1 tbs olive or sunflower oil
2 large onions, peeled and chopped
2 cloves garlic, crushed
100g/4oz/1$\frac{1}{2}$ cups mushrooms, chopped
4 large tomatoes, skinned and chopped
1 x 5ml sp/1 tsp tomato purée
50g/2oz/1 cup wholemeal breadcrumbs
2 x 15ml sp/2 tbs bran
25g/1oz/3 tbs blanched almonds, chopped
1 x 15ml sp/1 tbs fresh parsley, chopped
1 x 5ml sp/1 tsp lemon juice
salt and freshly ground black pepper
50g/2oz/$\frac{1}{2}$ cup vegetarian cheese, grated

1　Pierce the aubergines with a fork to prevent the skins from bursting, put them on a baking tray and bake them for 30 minutes at 350°F/ 180°C/gas mark 4, turning them once. Cut them in half lengthways and scoop out the flesh, leaving some to form thick skins for the shells. Chop the flesh.

2　Heat the oil in a pan and fry the onions and garlic over a moderate heat for 2 minutes, stirring occasionally. Add the mushrooms, tomatoes and tomato purée to the pan. Simmer for 5 minutes stirring occasionally, then add the chopped aubergine flesh, two-thirds of the breadcrumbs, half the bran, the almonds, parsley and lemon juice and season to taste with salt and freshly ground black pepper. Stir them all together well and simmer for 2–3 minutes.

3 Put the aubergine shells in an ovenproof dish and spoon the filling into the shells. Mix together the remaining breadcrumbs, bran and the cheese and sprinkle this over the tops of the aubergine shells, pressing down firmly on the filling. Bake for 20–25 minutes, until the cheese is bubbling and golden brown. Serve hot.

Leeks in Curry Dressing

▶ **CHO neg** ▶ **CALORIES 580**   *serves 4*

8 medium leeks, washed and cut into 15cm/5–6 inch lengths and
cooked until just tender

Dressing
3 x 15ml sp/3 tbs corn or sunflower oil
2 x 15ml sp/2 tbs wine vinegar
1 x 5ml sp/1 tsp curry powder
1 x 5ml sp/1 tsp made mustard
salt and freshly ground black pepper
pinch intense sweetener

1 Arrange the cooled leeks on 4 serving plates.
2 To make the dressing, put all the ingredients in a screw-top jar and
   shake well.
3 Pour the dressing over the leeks and chill until needed.

Courgettes à la Grecque

▶ CHO neg ▶ CALORIES 330 *serves 4*

2 x 15ml sp/2 tbs olive oil
1 onion, peeled and sliced
1–2 cloves garlic, crushed
450g/1 lb courgettes, sliced
1 x 15ml sp/1 tbs cider vinegar
2 x 15ml sp/2 tbs tomato purée
1 x 5ml sp/1 tsp thyme
6 x 15ml sp/6 tbs water
salt and freshly ground black pepper

1   Heat the oil in a pan and sauté the onion and garlic for 2–3 minutes. Add the courgettes and cook for 5 minutes, stirring occasionally. Add the vinegar, tomato purée, thyme, water and salt and freshly ground black pepper.

2   Mix all the ingredients together well. Bring them to the boil, cover and simmer for 15 minutes. Serve either hot or cold.

Mushrooms à la Grecque

▶ CHO neg ▶ CALORIES 410   *serves 4*

2 x 15ml sp/2 tbs olive oil
1 onion, peeled and chopped
1 clove garlic, crushed
4 tomatoes, skinned, seeded and finely chopped
450g/1 lb/6 cups button mushrooms, chopped
1 x 15ml sp/1 tbs tomato purée
1 wineglass dry white wine
2 x 15ml sp/2 tbs fresh parsley, chopped
salt and freshly ground black pepper

1   Heat the oil in a pan, add the onion and garlic and fry for 5 minutes. Then add the tomatoes and mushrooms and cook for 5 more minutes, stirring occasionally.

2   Stir in the tomato purée and wine. Bring to the boil then remove the pan from the heat immediately. Add all but 1 tbs of the parsley and season, stir well and leave the mixture to cool.

3   Chill for at least 2 hours before serving. Top with the reserved parsley before serving.

Summer Vegetable Salad

▶ CHO 20g ▶ CALORIES 540

serves 6

2 carrots, sliced
100g/4oz/1 cup broccoli, cooked *al dente*
100g/4oz/1 cup French beans, cooked *al dente*
100g/4oz/²⁄₃ cup sweetcorn, cooked
50g/2oz/¹⁄₃ cup lentils, cooked
2 courgettes, thinly sliced

Dressing

6 x 15ml sp/6 tbs reduced-calorie mayonnaise
bunch tarragon, chopped
2 x 15ml sp/2 tbs lemon juice
salt and freshly ground black pepper

1   Put all the vegetables into a salad bowl.
2   Mix all the dressing ingredients together then stir in to the vegetables until they are evenly coated with it. Adjust the seasoning to taste if necessary and chill until needed.

Cheese and Fruit Cocktail

▶ CHO 30g ▶ CALORIES 300   *serves 4*

2 red-skinned dessert apples, chopped (skins left on)
2 sticks celery, chopped
50g/2oz/¹/₂ cup reduced-fat cheese, diced
50g/2oz/¹/₃ cup grapes, halved and deseeded
1 orange, grated zest and juice of
2 x 15ml sp/2 tbs low-fat natural yogurt
a few lettuce leaves, shredded

1   Put the apples, celery, cheese and grapes into a bowl.
2   Mix the orange juice and yogurt together and add this to the bowl, mixing it together well with the fruit, vegetable and cheese.
3   Arrange the salad on a bed of lettuce and chill until you are ready to serve.

Stuffed Iceberg Lettuce

▶ CHO 20g ▶ CALORIES 510   *serves 4–6*

1 Iceberg lettuce
175g/6oz/³⁄₄ cup skimmed milk or low-fat soft cheese
1 x 15ml sp/1 tbs skimmed milk (if necessary)
1 red pepper, deseeded and finely diced
25g/1oz/2 tbs sultanas
25g/1oz/3 tbs walnuts, chopped
salt and freshly ground black pepper

1   Cut the top off the lettuce and reserve it. Using a sharp knife, scoop
    out the centre, leaving a 2.5cm/1 inch thick case. Chop the lettuce you
    scooped out and put it into a bowl.
2   Mix the soft cheese, milk, pepper, sultanas and walnuts together and
    season to taste with salt and freshly ground black pepper. Add half the
    chopped lettuce to this mixture and spoon it into the lettuce case and
    replace the lid.
3   Put the Stuffed Iceberg Lettuce on a serving plate and garnish with the
    remaining chopped lettuce. Keep it chilled until you are ready to
    serve.

Vegetable Rice

▶ **CHO 200g** ▶ **CALORIES 980**   *serves 4*

225g/8oz/1 cup long-grain rice
100g/4oz/²⁄₃ cup carrots, finely chopped
100g/4oz/²⁄₃ cup sweetcorn kernels
1 x 15ml sp/1 tbs parsley, finely chopped

1   Place the rice in a pan of boiling water. Cover and simmer for 15 minutes.
2   Add the vegetables and cook for a further 10 minutes or until the rice is tender.
3   Drain well, stir in the parsley and transfer to a warmed serving dish.

9 puddings and desserts

Almost everyone loves a good pudding or sophisticated dessert, whether it is hot or cold. What could be a better ending to a meal than a slice of cheesecake or a hearty crumble?

The recipes that follow use fruits that are high in fibre and a good source of vitamins, together with other high-fibre ingredients, such as wholemeal flour and dried fruits, and low-fat ingredients, such as low-fat spreads and dairy products. Where possible the virtually calorie-free artificial sweeteners are used instead of sugar to sweeten a dish and where sugar is used the quantities have been reduced as much as possible. All this means that you can eat a lovely dessert without feeling guilty – as long as you don't get too carried away!

Eve's Pudding

▶ CHO 170g ▶ CALORIES 1350

serves 8–10

450g/1 lb cooking apples, peeled, cored and sliced
1 orange, zest and juice of
1 lemon, zest and juice of
25g/1oz/3 tbs hazelnuts, finely chopped
2 x 15ml sp/2 tbs water

Topping
100g/4oz/$\frac{1}{2}$ cup low-fat spread
50g/2oz/$\frac{1}{3}$ cup caster sugar
2 size 3 eggs, beaten
100g/4oz/1 cup wholemeal self-raising flour
pinch baking powder
pinch cinnamon
1 x 15ml sp/1 tbs boiling water

1   Put the sliced apples in a deep 20 by 25cm/8 by 10 inch baking dish. Add the zest and juice of the orange and lemon, the nuts and water and mix them together well. Cover with foil and bake in the oven at 375°F/190°C/ gas mark 5 for 10–12 minutes.

2   Meanwhile, make the topping. Cream the low-fat spread and sugar together until the texture is light and fluffy. Add the beaten eggs gradually, beating the mixture well between each addition.

3   Gradually add the flour, folding it into the creamed mixture. Add the baking powder, cinnamon and water and mix them into the mixture. Spread the topping evenly over the fruit and return the dish to the oven for a further 25–30 minutes, or until the topping is well risen and springs back when touched. The pudding may be served hot or cold.

Baked Apples

▶ CHO 50g ▶ CALORIES 190   *serves 2*

2 medium cooking apples, cores removed
25g/1oz/2 tbs raisins
1 x 2.5ml sp/$^{1}/_{2}$ tsp ground cinnamon
1 x 2.5ml sp/$^{1}/_{2}$ tsp ground mixed spice

1   Slit the apple skins from top to bottom at intervals and then put them
    in an ovenproof dish. Mix the raisins with the spices and fill the core of
    each apple with the fruit mixture.
2   Cover the dish with foil and bake at 350°F/180°C/gas mark 4 for about
    30–40 minutes.

Bakewell Tart

▶ CHO 140g ▶ CALORIES 1350   *makes 8–10 portions*

Pastry

75g/3oz/¾ cup wholemeal flour
25g/1oz/¼ cup plain flour
pinch salt
25g/1oz/2 tbs low-fat spread
25g/1oz/2 tbs white polyunsaturated vegetable fat
cold water to mix

Filling

2 x 15ml sp/2 tbs pure fruit spread
50g/2oz/¼ cup low-fat spread
25g/1oz/2 tbs caster sugar
50g/2oz/¼ cup ground rice
25g/1oz/¼ cup ground almonds
1 size 3 egg, beaten
few drops almond essence (optional)
blanched almonds to decorate

1 Make the pastry by sieving the two flours and salt together into a bowl, cutting in the fats until they are well mixed with the flour and then stirring in a little cold water at a time until the mixture forms a smooth, pliable dough, neither too hard nor too soft. Line an 18cm/7 inch fluted flan ring with the pastry, saving the oddments left over. Spread the pure fruit spread over the bottom.

2 Now make the filling. Cream the low-fat spread and sugar until the mixture becomes light and fluffy. Mix together the ground rice and ground almonds and add this to the creamed mixture with the beaten egg and almond essence (if using), combining all the ingredients together well. Spread the mixture over the jam.

3 Knead the reserved scraps of pastry together, roll it out and cut it into strips. Decorate the top of the tart by making a lattice pattern with the strips and dotting with blanched almonds.

4 Bake the tart at 375°F/190°C/gas mark 5 for 30–35 minutes.

Peach Pudding

▶ CHO 130g ▶ CALORIES 1120   *serves 10*

75g/3oz/$^1/_3$ cup low-fat spread
50g/2oz/$^1/_3$ cup caster sugar
2 size 3 eggs, beaten
50g/2oz/$^1/_2$ cup wholemeal self-raising flour
25g/1oz/$^1/_4$ cup ground almonds
1 x 5ml sp/1 tsp ground cinnamon
3 fresh peaches, peeled, stoned and sliced
2 x 5ml sp/2 tsp demerara sugar

1   Cream the low-fat spread and sugar until the mixture has become pale. Beat in the eggs a little at a time alternately with the flour, ground almonds and half the cinnamon. Spoon the mixture into a lightly greased 23cm/9 inch round, shallow ovenproof dish or pie plate. Arrange the peach slices over the mixture and push them into it.

2   Mix the remaining cinnamon with the demerara sugar and sprinkle it over the pudding, then bake it at 375°F/190°C/gas mark 5 for approximately 30 minutes or until it has cooked. The mixture should have risen, be golden brown and the sugar should have caramelized.

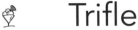

Trifle

▶ CHO 110g ▶ CALORIES 1040   *serves 6*

1 x 425g/15oz can/2 cups fruit cocktail in natural juice
1 packet sugar-free jelly crystals
2 x 15ml sp/2 tbs custard powder
275ml/$\frac{1}{2}$ pint/1$\frac{1}{3}$ cups skimmed milk
intense artificial sweetener to taste
150ml/$\frac{1}{4}$ pint carton/$\frac{2}{3}$ cup whipping cream, whipped
a few flaked almonds, toasted

1 Drain the fruit and reserve the juice. Arrange the fruit in the bottom of
   a bowl.
2 Make up the jelly crystals according to the directions on the packet
   and make up to 550ml/1 pint using the reserved fruit juice. Pour the
   jelly onto the fruit and leave to set.
3 Make the custard according to the directions on the tin and sweeten if
   necessary. Pour it over the fruit and top with the whipped cream and
   toasted almonds.
4 Chill the trifle well before serving.

Raspberry and Kiwi Whip

▶ CHO 10g ▶ CALORIES 380   *serves 4–6*

100g/4oz/¹⁄₂ cup quark or skimmed milk cheese
1 x 150g/5fl oz carton/²⁄₃ cup low-fat natural yogurt
225g/8oz/2 cups raspberries, fresh or frozen, puréed
intense artificial sweetener to taste
2 kiwi fruit, peeled and sliced

1   Mix the soft cheese and yogurt together in a bowl. Add the raspberry
    purée and sweetener to taste.
2   Arrange the kiwi fruit in individual dishes or 1 large bowl, reserving
    2 or 3 slices. Pour the raspberry mixture over the fruit and chill in a
    refrigerator before serving. Then decorate with the reserved kiwi fruit
    slices.

Yogurt Gooseberry Fool

▶ CHO 10g ▶ CALORIES 160   *serves 6*

450g/1 lb gooseberries, topped and tailed
intense artificial sweetener to taste
1 x 150g/5fl oz carton/²⁄₃ cup low-fat natural yogurt or diet
    gooseberry yogurt
1–2 drops green food colouring (optional)

1   Put the gooseberries in a pan with a little water and cook them gently
    until the fruit is soft. Purée the gooseberries in a blender and press
    through a sieve to remove the seeds. Fold the yogurt into the fruit
    purée. Add 1–2 drops of green food colouring if using.

2   Divide the fool between 6 individual glass dessert bowls or wine gob-
    lets and chill until you are ready to serve.

▶   *Note to Cooks Because each portion will have an insignificant amount
of CHO, it does not have to be counted in the diet.*

Fruit and Yogurt Whips

▶ **CHO 60g** ▶ **CALORIES 410**   *serves 4*

1 banana, peeled and chopped
1 x 5ml sp/1 tsp lemon juice
2 size 3 egg whites
1 x 15ml sp//1 tbs intense artificial sweetener
2 x 150g/5fl oz cartons/$\frac{2}{3}$ cup low-fat natural yogurt
25g/1oz/2 tbs dried mixed fruit
25g/1oz/3 tbs chopped hazelnuts

1   Mix the banana with the lemon juice in a bowl to prevent it browning.
2   Whisk the egg whites until they are stiff, then gently fold in the sweetener and yogurt using a metal spoon.
3   Fold in the dried fruit and nuts, reserving a little to decorate the whips.
4   Divide the mixture between 4 dishes and sprinkle each one with the reserved nuts. Serve immediately.

▶ *Note to Cooks Try using a diet fruit-flavoured yogurt instead of the natural yogurt, say, apple and cinnamon, peach or apricot.*

Yogurt Snow with Raspberry Sauce

▶ CHO 20g ▶ CALORIES 160 *serves 3–4*

2 x 150g/5fl oz cartons/1 cup low-fat natural yogurt
intense artificial sweetener to taste
1 egg white, beaten until stiff

Raspberry sauce
100g/4oz/1 cup raspberries
1 lemon, juice of
intense artificial sweetener to taste
a few mint leaves to decorate

1 Drain the yogurt in a muslin-lined sieve for several hours (preferably overnight). Add the sweetener to the drained yogurt and fold in the beaten egg white. Spoon the Snow into ramekin dishes and chill for about an hour.

2 Meanwhile, purée the raspberries – reserving 3 or 4 to decorate – in a liquidizer for several minutes. Add the lemon juice and sweetener and purée again. Strain the sauce into a serving jug.

3 Decorate the Snow with the reserved raspberries and the mint leaves and serve the sauce in a jug for people to help themselves.

▶ *Note to Cooks You can use a clean 'all-purpose cloth' if you don't happen to have any muslin.*

Apple Delight

▶ CHO 50g ▶ CALORIES 260   *serves 2*

2 x 150g/5fl oz cartons/²/₃ cup low-fat natural yogurt
2 eating apples, peeled, cored and grated
¹/₂ lemon, zest and juice of
intense artificial sweetener to taste (optional)
2 walnut halves to decorate

1   Pour the yogurt into a bowl. Add the apple, lemon zest and juice and
    sweeten to taste.
2   Pour the Delight into 2 individual dishes and chill well before serving.
3   Top each dish with a walnut half and serve.

Raspberry Mousse

▶ CHO 39.99g ▶ CALORIES 376   *serves 6–8*

1 sachet raspberry sugar-free jelly crystals
1 x 400g/14oz can/2 cups raspberries in natural juice
2 size 3 egg whites
1 x 150ml/5fl oz carton/²⁄₃ cup fromage frais

1   Make the jelly up to 275ml/¹⁄₂ pint with boiling water.
2   Purée the raspberries and make up to 275ml/¹⁄₂ pint with water (sieve it to remove the pips if you prefer a smooth texture).
3   Add the raspberry mixture to the jelly and, once it has cooled, put it in the refrigerator until it has nearly set – until the jelly coats the back of a spoon (this usually takes about 1 hour).
4   Whisk the cream until it is thick and stir the fromage frais into the jelly mixture. Beat the egg whites until they are stiff and gently fold them into the jelly using a metal spoon.
5   Pour the mousse into a dish and leave it to set in the refrigerator.

Note to Cooks *An individual/single serving would have a negligible amount of CHO.*

Marbled Apricots

▶ CHO 40g ▶ CALORIES 240   *serves 4–6*

450g/1 lb/2 cups fresh apricots, cut in half and the stones removed
200g/7oz/1 cup fat-free fromage frais
intense artificial sweetener to taste (optional)

1   Stew the apricots in a little water until they are tender. Leave them to cool then purée them in a blender or food processor.
2   Pour the fromage frais into a 500ml/1 pint glass bowl, add the sweetener, if using, spoon in the apricot purée and blend only until a marble effect occurs – do not mix them together thoroughly.
3   Chill the mixture before serving.

Pears Cassis

▶ CHO 80g ▶ CALORIES 320   *serves 4*

4 pears, peeled, cored and halved

275ml/$^{1}/_{2}$ pint/1$^{1}/_{3}$ cups water

1 vanilla pod or

2–3 drops vanilla essence

275g/10oz can/1$^{1}/_{2}$ cups blackcurrants in natural juice

intense artificial sweetener to taste

2 x 5ml sp/2 tsp arrowroot

1   Put the pear halves in a pan with the water and vanilla. Cover the pan, bring to the boil, then simmer until the pears look almost transparent (this will take about 20–30 minutes).

2   Meanwhile, purée the blackcurrants.

3   When the pears are ready, drain them, reserving the cooking liquid, put them in a serving dish and keep them warm.

4   Make the blackcurrant purée up to 425ml/¾ pint with the reserved liquid from the pears, adding sweetener to taste, and heat it gently.

5   Mix the arrowroot with 2 tbs of the pear liquid and add it to the pan, stirring as you do so and until it thickens slightly, then pour it over the pears and serve.

Cheesecake

▶ CHO 140g ▶ CALORIES 1600   *serves 6–8*

50g/2oz/$^1\!/_4$ cup low-fat spread
175g/6oz/1$^1\!/_2$ cups wholemeal biscuits, crushed
1 sachet gelatine
1 orange, finely grated rind and juice of
225g/8oz/1 cup skimmed milk cheese, quark or low-fat soft cheese
1 x 150g/5fl oz carton/$^2\!/_3$ cup low-fat natural yogurt
liquid sweetener to taste
2 size 3 eggs, separated
100g/4oz/1 cup fresh or frozen raspberries

1   Melt the low-fat spread and mix it with the crushed biscuits. Press it
    down evenly in the bottom of an 18cm/7 inch spring release or a loose
    bottomed tin. Leave it to chill in the refrigerator for 30 minutes.

2   Meanwhile, dissolve gelatine in 3 tbs of hot water. Put the orange rind
    and juice and skimmed milk cheese or quark into a bowl. Add the
    yogurt, sweetener and egg yolks and mix them together well. Add the
    cooled gelatine and mix well. Whisk the egg whites until they are stiff
    and then lightly fold them into the yogurt mixture. Carefully pour the
    mixture into the tin, smooth the top and chill for several hours, prefer-
    ably overnight.

3   Remove the cheesecake from the tin, leaving the base in place, and
    put it on a flat serving plate. Decorate the top with the raspberries.

▶ *Note to Cooks You can freeze the cheesecake if you wish, but do so
before putting the fruit on top and decorate it instead when you defrost it
to use at a later date.*

Fresh Fruit Jelly

▶ CHO 40g ▶ CALORIES 190　　　　　　　*serves 6–8*

1 packet sugar-free jelly crystals
1 red apple, cored and sliced
1 orange, peeled and segmented
20 grapes (10 black and 10 white)
You can use any fresh fruit you like that is in season. Strawberries,
　bananas, tangerines and white grapes are all good alternatives.

1　Make up the jelly crystals according to the directions on the packet.
2　Put the fruit into a bowl and pour the jelly over it. Leave it to cool then
　chill it until it has set in a refrigerator before serving.

Peach Ice-Cream

▶ CHO 70g ▶ CALORIES 500   *serves 6–8*

1 x 425g/15oz can/2 cups peach slices in natural juice
1 x 150g/5fl oz carton/²⁄₃ cup low-fat natural yogurt
1 x 170g/6–7oz can/³⁄₄ cup evaporated milk, well chilled

1   Put the peaches and the juice into a blender or food processor and
    blend for 1–2 minutes.
2   Whisk the evaporated milk until it is thick and has doubled in volume.
    Whisk in the yogurt and gently fold the peach purée into the mixture.
3   Pour it into a freezer-proof container and freeze it until it has frozen
    around the edges (this takes about 1–2 hours). Beat the mixture break-
    ing up the crystals and pour it back into the container or individual
    cartons and freeze it uncovered.
4   Put the ice-cream in a refrigerator for 10–15 minutes to soften a little
    before you serve it.

Fruit Fool

▶ CHO 50g ▶ CALORIES 280   *serves 2*

175g/6oz/1 cup blackcurrants
4 x 5ml sp/4 tsp custard powder
150ml/¼ pint/²⁄₃ cup skimmed milk
1 x 150g/5fl oz carton/²⁄₃ cup low-fat natural yogurt
1 x 5ml sp/1 tsp intense artificial sweetener

1   Cook the blackcurrants in approximately 2 tbs water until they are soft, then sieve or liquidize the fruit.

2   Make the custard by mixing the custard powder with 4 tsp of the milk, warming the rest of the milk, mixing in the custard powder mixture and stirring continuously until it thickens, then take it off the heat and leave it to cool.

3   When the custard has cooled, add the puréed fruit and yogurt to the custard and mix them together thoroughly. Sweeten the fool to taste and chill before serving.

Grape Jelly

▶ CHO 30g ▶ CALORIES 190   *serves 6*

150ml/¼ pint/⅔ cup unsweetened white grape juice
generous 3 x 15ml sp/3 tbs lemon juice
275ml/½ pint/1⅓ cups water
15g/½ oz/1 tbs gelatine, dissolved in 3 tbs cold water
artificial sweetener to taste
75g/3oz/½ cup small black or green grapes, halved and depipped

1   Pour the grape and lemon juice and water into a dish. Add the dissolved gelatine, stirring, then chill the jelly until the mixture has the consistency of unbeaten egg white.
2   Stir in the grapes and chill until the jelly has set.

Pears in Mulled Wine

▶ CHO 60g ▶ CALORIES 430   *serves 4*

4 ripe even-sized pears
275ml/$\frac{1}{2}$ pint/$1\frac{1}{3}$ cups red wine
pinch grated nutmeg
1 stick cinnamon
$\frac{1}{2}$ lemon, rind of
few drops lemon juice
4 cloves
intense artificial sweetener to taste

1   Peel the pears, leaving the stalks on. Slice a sliver off the bottom so that they will stand up.
2   Put all the ingredients, except the pears, into a saucepan and heat for 5 minutes. Pour everything into a small, deep-sided dish and stand the pears in it, basting them with the wine mixture.
3   Bake the pears at 350°F/180°C/gas mark 4 for 30 minutes, basting them occasionally.
4   Serve the pears immediately, with a little of the cooking juices dribbled over them.

Summer Pudding

▶ CHO 90g ▶ CALORIES 610   *serves 6*

675g/1½–2 lb mixed soft fruits, such as blackcurrants, redcurrants,
**   raspberries and blackberries**
intense artificial sweetener to taste
about 6 slices of stale white bread, crusts removed

1   Put the soft fruits in a saucepan and cook them gently for 5 minutes or
    until the juices run and the fruits soften and sweeten to taste.
2   Meanwhile, line the bottom and sides of a 825ml/1½ pint pudding
    basin with the bread, ensuring that there are no gaps between the
    slices and reserving 1½ slices for the top.
3   Put the fruit and all but 2 x 15ml sp/2 tbs of the juice into the bread-
    lined basin, cover with the reserved bread. Put a plate over the top
    and weigh it down with weights or a heavy tin. Chill the pudding
    overnight.
4   To unmould the pudding, hold the serving plate, inverted, over the
    top of the basin and turn the pudding over. Pour the reserved fruit
    juice over the pudding just before serving.

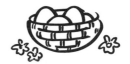

10 home baking

Home-baked bread and teatime treats are pleasures that shouldn't be a thing of the past. You can still enjoy them if you like to treat yourself occasionally. They needn't take long to make either and beat bought versions hands down.

The recipes for traditional favourites here have been modified so that high-fibre, low-fat and low-sugar ingredients are used. Try some with your afternoon tea today!

Wholemeal Bread

▶ **CHO 580g** ▶ **CALORIES 2990**   *makes 3 450g/1lb loaves*

900g/2 lb/8 cups wholemeal flour
1 x 15ml sp/1 tbs salt
50g/2oz/¼ cup low-fat spread
1 x 15ml sp/1 tbs easy-blend dried yeast
1 x 15ml sp/1 tbs malt extract
550ml/1 pint/2½ cups tepid water

1   Combine the flour, salt and yeast, then rub in the low-fat spread.
    Dissolve the yeast and the malt in the water and gradually add it to the
    flour, mixing it in well. Knead it to a soft dough, then turn it out onto a
    floured board and knead for 10–15 minutes until it is smooth and elastic.
2   Divide the mixture into 3 and put each in a lightly oiled 450g/1 lb loaf
    tin. Put them in a warm place to prove (double in size).
3   Bake them at 400°F/200°C/gas mark 6 for 10 minutes then reduce the
    temperature to 350°F/180°C/gas mark 4 for 25–35 minutes. You can
    tell that they are done if when you turn them out they sound hollow
    when you rap the bottoms. Turn them out of the tins and leave them
    to cool on a wire rack.

▶ **Note to cooks** *These loaves freeze well wrapped in foil once they have
cooled.*

Victoria Sandwich

▶ CHO 120g ▶ CALORIES 1060   *serves 8*

100g/4oz/^{1}/$_2$ cup low-fat spread
50g/2oz/^{1}/$_3$ cup caster sugar
2 size 3 eggs, lightly beaten
1 x 15ml sp/1 tbs hot water
100g/4oz/1 cup self-raising wholemeal flour
pinch baking powder

1   Cream the low-fat spread and sugar together until the mixture is light
     and creamy. Beat in the eggs and water. Sieve the flour and baking
     powder into another bowl, then gradually add it to the creamed mix-
     ture, folding it in so that they are thoroughly mixed together.

2   Divide the mixture between 2 15cm/6 inch, lightly greased sandwich
     tins and bake at 350°F/180°C/gas mark 4 for 20–25 minutes until they
     have risen well, spring back when touched and are golden brown. Turn
     them out onto a wire tray to cool.

3   You can then fill the cake with pure fruit spread and whipped cream
     and sprinkle a little powdered intense sweetener over the top or fill it
     with pure fruit spread and some of the Butter Icing recipe on page
     199. A pretty finishing touch is to lay a paper doily on top of the filled
     cake and sift a little powdered sweetener over it. When you lift the
     doily, there will be a lacy pattern.

▶ *Note to cooks If you use jam in the cake remember to add the CHO
and calories. 1 oz pure fruit spread contains approx. 10g CHO, 35 cals. If
using whipped cream a 142ml/5fl oz carton contains 510 calories.*

Fairy Cakes

▶ CHO 90g ▶ CALORIES 660 *makes 10*

50g/2oz/¼ cup low-fat spread
25g/1oz/2 tbs caster sugar
1 size 3 egg, beaten
50g/2oz/½ cup self-raising wholemeal flour
50g/2oz/⅓ cup raisins
1 x 15ml sp/1 tbs boiling water, if needed

1   Cream the low-fat spread and sugar together until the mixture pales in colour. Add half the beaten egg and 1 x 5ml sp/1 tsp of the flour and beat well. Add the remaining egg and 1 x 5ml sp/1 tsp of the flour and beat well. Add the remaining flour gradually and the raisins, folding them in gently using a metal spoon. The mixture should now be of a dropping consistency (if it is not, add the 1 x 15ml sp/1 tbs of boiling water).

2   Spoon equal amounts of the mixture into 10 paper cases in a patty tin and bake on the middle shelf of the oven for 10–15 minutes at 350°F/180°C/gas mark 4 until the Fairy Cakes have risen well, are golden brown and firm to the touch.

Butterfly Cakes

▶ CHO 120g ▶ CALORIES 1160 *makes 12–15*

1 Victoria Sandwich recipe (see page 183)
a little granular intense artificial sweetener
Butter Icing recipe (see page 199) flavoured with 1–2 drops vanilla
essence

1   Prepare the Victoria Sandwich recipe as given on page 183 and divide
    the mixture between 12–15 paper cases in patty tins. Bake them in a
    350°F/180°C/gas mark 4 oven for 12–15 minutes until the cakes have
    risen and are golden brown. Remove them from the tin and leave them
    to cool on a wire rack.
2   Meanwhile, prepare the Butter Icing as given on page 199.
3   When the cakes have cooled, cut a slice from the top of each bun and
    put a tsp of the Butter Icing over the cut cake. Cut the removed slices
    in half and place them on the cakes, angling them into the Butter Icing
    to form 'wings'. Dust the cakes with granular intense artificial sweet-
    ener. The cakes are tastiest when they are fresh.

Banana and Walnut Slices

▶ **CHO 160g** ▶ **CALORIES 1580** *makes 16*

100g/4oz/¹⁄₂ cup low-fat spread
50g/2oz/¹⁄₃ cup sugar
2 size 3 eggs
100g/4oz/1 cup wholemeal self-raising flour
1 x 5ml sp/1 tsp baking powder
2 small bananas, mashed
75g/3oz/²⁄₃ cup walnuts, chopped

1   Preheat the oven to 375°F/190°C/gas mark 5.
2   Cream the low-fat spread and the sugar together until the mixture is
     light and fluffy. Beat in the eggs, one at a time, adding a tbs of the
     flour with the second egg. Fold in the remaining flour and the baking
     powder together with the bananas.
3   Spread the mixture evenly in a lined and greased 15 by 25cm/6 by 10
     inch shallow tin and sprinkle the walnuts over the top. Bake in the pre-
     heated oven for 20–25 minutes.
4   When the mixture has cooked, leave it in the tin but cut it into 16 equal
     pieces. Leave the tin on a wire rack to cool, then turn the slices out and
     store them in an airtight container.

Tea Bread

▶ CHO 210g ▶ CALORIES 1680   *makes 1 450g/1lb loaf*

100g/4oz/$\frac{1}{2}$ cup low-fat spread
50g/2oz/$\frac{1}{3}$ cup caster sugar
1 size 3 egg, beaten
2 small bananas, mashed
1 x 150g/5fl oz carton/$\frac{2}{3}$ cup low-fat natural yogurt
50g/2oz/$\frac{1}{2}$ cup white self-raising flour
100g/4oz/1 cup wholemeal self-raising flour
50g/2oz/$\frac{1}{2}$ cup walnuts, chopped
25g/1oz/2 tbs sultanas

1   Cream the low-fat spread and sugar until the mixture is light and fluffy. Add the egg and beat it in well. Stir in the bananas and yogurt. Gently fold in the flour, walnuts and sultanas.

2   Spoon the mixture into a lightly greased 450g/1 lb loaf tin and bake at 375°F/190°C/gas mark 5 for approximately 1 hour or until it is cooked (check it by inserting a clean skewer into the centre and leaving it there for a couple of seconds – if it comes out clean, the Tea Bread is done).

Rhubarb and Raisin Cake

▶ **CHO 210g** ▶ **CALORIES 1260**　　　　*makes 12 portions*

225g/8oz/$^1/_2$ lb rhubarb, chopped
50g/2oz/$^1/_4$ cup low-fat spread
225g/8oz/2 cups self-raising wholemeal flour
1 x 5ml sp/1 tsp baking powder
100g/4oz/$^2/_3$ cup raisins
1 size 3 egg, beaten
4 x 15ml sp/4 tbs skimmed milk

1　Cook the rhubarb in a little water for 5–10 minutes.
2　Rub the low-fat spread into the flour and baking powder, which you
　　have sieved together into a bowl. Add the rhubarb and raisins and mix
　　them in. Add the egg and milk and mix them in well.
3　Pour the mixture into a lightly oiled 18cm/7 inch cake tin and bake at
　　375°F/190°C/gas mark 5 for 1 hour. Turn the cake out and leave it to
　　cool on a wire rack.

▶ **Note to cooks** *This cake freezes well. Just wrap it in foil once it has
cooled.*

Celebration Cake

▶ CHO 320g ▶ CALORIES 2300   *makes 12 portions*

25g/1oz/2 tbs sugar
75g/3oz/^{1}/$_2$ cup sultanas
75g/3oz/^{1}/$_2$ cup currants
75g/3oz/^{1}/$_2$ cup raisins
300ml/^{1}/$_2$ pint/1^1/$_3$ cups Guinness
50g/2oz/^{1}/$_4$ cup low-fat spread
225g/8oz/2 cups 100 per cent wholemeal flour
1 x 2.5ml sp/^{1}/$_2$ cup tsp baking powder
1 x 5ml sp/1 tsp mixed spice
75g/3oz/^{2}/$_3$ cup walnuts, chopped
3 size 3 eggs, beaten

1   Put the sugar, fruit and Guinness in a pan, bring it to the boil, then
    leave it to simmer for 20 minutes. Add the low-fat spread and leave it
    to cool. Add the beaten egg to the mixture. Sieve the flour and baking
    powder together into a bowl, then stir it into the pan.

2   Pour the mixture into a well-oiled 18cm/7 inch square tin and bake at
    350°F/180°C/gas mark 4 for 1–1^1/$_2$ hours. Leave it to cool in the tin on
    a wire rack.

3   To test whether the cake is cooked, insert a clean skewer into the
    centre and leave it there for 2 seconds. If the skewer if clean when you
    pull it out, the cake is done.

▶ ***Note to cooks*** *This cake freezes well wrapped in foil.*

Date and Walnut Loaf

▶ CHO 370g ▶ CALORIES 2290   *makes 1 900g/2 lb loaf*

225g/8oz/1$\frac{1}{3}$ cups stoned dates, chopped
1 x 2.5ml sp/$\frac{1}{2}$ tsp bicarbonate of soda
1 x 2.5ml sp/$\frac{1}{2}$ tsp salt
150ml/$\frac{1}{4}$ pint/$\frac{2}{3}$ cup boiling water
100g/4oz/$\frac{1}{2}$ cup low-fat spread
75g/3oz/$\frac{1}{2}$ cup brown sugar
1 size 3 egg, beaten
225g/8oz/2 cups wholemeal self-raising flour
50g/2oz/$\frac{1}{2}$ cup walnuts, chopped

1   Put the dates, bicarbonate of soda and salt in a basin, pour the boiling water over them and put to one side.
2   Meanwhile, cream the low-fat spread and sugar and beat in the egg. Stir in flour, nuts and date mixture and stir until all the ingredients are combined. Pour the mixture into a lightly greased 900g/2 lb loaf tin and bake at 350°F/180°C/gas mark 4 for 1–1$\frac{1}{2}$ hours. To test whether the loaf is done, poke a clean skewer into the centre of it, leave it there for 2 seconds, then if it comes out clean, it is done.
3   Then turn it out onto a wire rack and leave it to cool. When it has cooled, store in an airtight container.

Prune and Nut Cake

▶ **CHO 190g** ▶ **CALORIES 1310**   *makes 12 portions*

225g/8oz/2 cups self-raising wholemeal flour
pinch salt
1 x 5ml sp/1 tsp grated nutmeg
1 small orange, grated zest of
25g/1oz/2 tbs low-fat spread
50g/2oz/¹/₂ cup walnuts, chopped
75g/3oz/³/₄ cup stoneless prunes, chopped
1 size 3 egg, beaten
100ml/3fl oz/¹/₃ cup skimmed milk
3 x 15ml sp/3 tbs juice from the orange

1   Sieve the flour, salt and spices into a bowl and add the orange zest.
     Mix in the low-fat spread using a fork. Stir in the walnuts and prunes
     and beat in the egg, milk and orange juice until everything is well
     mixed.
2   Turn the mixture into a greased 15cm/6 inch round cake tin and bake
     at 375°F/190°C/gas mark 5 for 40–45 minutes or until the cake is well
     risen and golden brown and a skewer pierced through the centre of
     the cake comes out clean.
3   Allow it to cool before serving.

▶ **Note to cooks** Serve this with Curd Cheese Topping (see page 198)
for a special occasion.

Rock Cakes

▶ CHO 230g ▶ CALORIES 1460   *makes 14*

100g/4oz/1 cup self-raising wholemeal flour
100g/4oz/1 cup self-raising white flour
100g/4oz/$\frac{1}{2}$ cup low-fat spread
50g/2oz/$\frac{1}{3}$ cup granulated sugar
50g/2oz/$\frac{1}{3}$ cup currants
1 size 3 egg, beaten
75ml/$\frac{1}{8}$ pint/$\frac{1}{4}$ cup skimmed milk

1   Sieve the flours into a mixing bowl. Rub the low-fat spread into the flours until the mixture resembles fine breadcrumbs. Then stir in the sugar and currants.

2   Make a well in the centre and pour the beaten egg and milk into it. Mix all the ingredients together, stirring round in the well, gradually incorporating all the dry ingredients.

3   Make 14 even-sized mounds of the mixture on a greased baking sheet and bake at 400°F/200°C/gas mark 6 for 10–15 minutes.

4   Leave the Rock Cakes to cool on a wire rack before serving them.

Maids of Honour

▶ CHO 200g ▶ CALORIES 1570   *makes 15–16*

Pastry

100g/4oz/1 cup wholemeal flour
50g/2oz/$^1/_2$ cup white flour
pinch salt
50g/2oz/$^1/_4$ cup low-fat spread
25g/1oz/2 tbs white polyunsaturated vegetable fat
a little cold water to mix

Filling

8 x 5ml sp/8 tsp pure fruit spread
50g/2oz/$^1/_4$ cup low-fat spread
25g/1oz/2 tbs caster sugar
1 size 3 egg, beaten
50g/2oz/$^1/_2$ cup self-raising wholemeal flour

1   Make the pastry by sieving the flours and salt into a bowl and rubbing the fats into the flour and stirring a little cold water into the mixture to bind it together.

2   Refrigerate the pastry for 30 minutes, then roll it out and, using a 7cm/3 inch round pastry cutter, cut out 15–16 shapes and put them in lightly greased patty tins. Put a half teaspoonful of the pure fruit spread in the bottom of each.

3   Cream the low-fat spread and sugar until the mixture is creamy, then fold in the beaten egg and flour. Put a small spoonful of the mixture in each case and bake them at 400°F/200°C/gas mark 6 for 15–20 minutes.

4   Leave them to cool on a wire rack.

Madeleines

▶ CHO 150g ▶ CALORIES 1760   *makes 10*

1 Victoria Sandwich recipe (see page 183)
75g/3oz/$^1/_4$ cup reduced-sugar raspberry jam, warmed
100g/4oz/1$^1/_3$ cups desiccated coconut
5 glacé cherries, halved
angelica leaves to decorate

1   Make the Victoria Sandwich mixture as given on page 183.
2   Spoon the mixture into 10 lightly greased dariole moulds so that they
    are ⅔ full and bake at 350°F/ 180°C/gas mark 4 for approximately 15
    minutes or until the mixture has risen and turned golden brown.
3   Loosen the madeleines round the edges with a knife and turn them
    out onto a cooling rack. When they are cool, thinly spread the jam over
    them and roll them in the coconut until they are coated in it. Put a
    glacé cherry on top of each cake and angelica leaves each side of it.

Jam Tarts

▶ **CHO 130g** ▶ **CALORIES 890**

makes 18–20

75g/3oz/³⁄₄ cup wholemeal flour
25g/1oz/¹⁄₄ cup plain flour
25g/1oz/2 tbs low-fat spread
25g/1oz/2 tbs white polyunsaturated vegetable fat
2 x 15ml sp/2 tbs cold water
1 x 5ml sp/1 tsp polyunsaturated oil
6–6¹⁄₂ x 15ml sp/6–6¹⁄₂ tbs reduced-sugar jam

1 Make the pastry by sieving the flours together into a bowl, rubbing the fats into the flours until the mixture resembles fine breadcrumbs, then adding the water and oil and working the mixture into a dough.

2 Chill the pastry for 30 minutes before rolling it out on a lightly floured surface. Using a 5cm/2 inch pastry cutter, cut out 18–20 rounds, gathering the scraps together and rolling it out again as necessary to use up as much of the pastry as possible.

3 Put the pastry circles in lightly greased patty tins and put a teaspoonful of jam into each. Bake for 15–20 minutes at 400°F/200°C/gas mark 6. Cool them on a wire rack.

Cinnamon Scone

▶ CHO 170g ▶ CALORIES 1100

serves 8–10

225g/8oz/2 cups self-raising wholemeal flour
pinch salt
2 x 5ml sp/2 tsp baking powder
3 x 5ml sp/3 tsp cinnamon
50g/2oz/$\frac{1}{4}$ cup low-fat spread
1 x 15ml sp/1 tbs caster sugar
1 size 3 egg, lightly beaten
about 150ml/$\frac{1}{4}$ pint/$\frac{2}{3}$ cup skimmed milk
1 x 5ml sp/1 tsp intense artificial sweetener

1   Sieve the flour, salt, baking powder and 2 tsp of the cinnamon into a bowl and rub in the low-fat spread until the mixture resembles fine breadcrumbs.
2   Stir in the sugar then gradually pour in the egg and milk and stir the mixture until it forms a soft dough. Turn it onto a floured surface, knead it gently until it is smooth, then roll the dough out into a round approximately 18cm/7 inch in diameter and 2.5cm/1 inch thick.
3   Put the scone on a lightly greased baking sheet and score it into 8 portions. Brush the surface with milk and sprinkle the remaining cinnamon over the top. Bake it at 425°F/220°C/gas mark 7 for 15–20 minutes until the scone has risen and is firm to the touch.
4   Sprinkle the intense artificial sweetener over the scone once it comes out of the oven.

Rich Scones

▶ CHO 210g ▶ CALORIES 1230　　　　　　*makes 12–14*

225g/8oz/2 cups self-raising wholemeal flour
1 x 2.5ml sp/$^1/_2$ tsp salt
50g/2oz/$^1/_4$ cup low-fat spread
25g/1oz/2 tbs sugar
50g/2oz/$^1/_3$ cup sultanas
1 size 3 egg, beaten with sufficient skimmed milk to make it up to
　　150ml/$^1/_4$ pint/$^2/_3$ cup

1　Sieve the flour and salt together into a bowl and rub the low-fat spread
　into them. Stir in the sugar and sultanas. Add the egg and milk, reserv-
　ing enough to glaze the tops later.

2　Knead the resulting dough lightly on a floured surface and roll it out to
　an even 2.5cm/1 inch thickness. Using a 5cm/2 inch pastry cutter, cut
　out as many rounds as you can, gathering together the scraps and
　rolling it out again to use as much of the dough as you can.

3　Put them on a lightly greased baking sheet and brush the tops with the
　reserved liquid. Bake them in a hot oven at 425°F/220°C/gas mark 7
　for approximately 10 minutes, then cool them on a wire rack.

Curd Cheese Topping

▶ CHO neg ▶ CALORIES 130   *sufficient for a 18cm/7inch cake*

75g/3oz/$\frac{1}{3}$ cup curd cheese
liquid intense artificial sweetener to taste
flavouring and/or colouring (optional)

1   Beat the curd cheese until it is smooth and fairly soft.
2   Add the sweetener to taste and colouring or flavouring if liked.

▶ *Note to cooks Use the topping just to sandwich cakes together or to decorate the top as well.*

Butter Icing

▶ CHO neg ▶ CALORIES 100   *sufficient for 6 small cakes*

2 x 15ml sp/2 tbs powdered intense artificial sweetener
25g/1oz/2 tbs low-fat spread

1   Beat the ingredients together to form a smooth paste, shortly before
     you intend using it.

▶   ***Note to cooks*** *This versatile icing can be flavoured in a variety of ways
depending on what you like and the cake you are decorating. Try a few
drops of vanilla essence or a tablespoon of cocoa powder or a teaspoon of
coffee essence.*

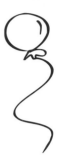

11 festive occasions

Festive times need not be a time of denial. Try these tasty adaptations of traditional favourites and you'll be doing yourself good without you or your guests even noticing. You can feel confident that at Christmas, especially, a time when good food is at the centre of all the festivities, you, your family and friends can all enjoy a feast of *good* things – in all senses of the word.

Broccoli and Mushroom Flan

▶ CHO 110g ▶ CALORIES 1710   *serves 6–8*

Pastry

100g/4oz/1 cup wholemeal flour
50g/2oz/$^1/_2$ cup plain flour
pinch salt
50g/2oz/$^1/_4$ cup low-fat spread
25g/1oz/2 tbs white polyunsaturated vegetable fat
a little cold water to bind

Filling

225g/8oz/2 cups broccoli cut into small florets
100g/4oz/1$^1/_2$ cups mushrooms, sliced
1 clove garlic, crushed
100g/4oz/1 cup reduced-fat cheddar cheese, grated
2 size 3 eggs, lightly beaten
1 x 150g/5fl oz carton/$^2/_3$ cup single cream
salt and freshly ground black pepper

1   Make the pastry first. Sieve the flours and salt into a bowl. Rub the fats
    into the flours until the mixture resembles fine breadcrumbs, then mix
    in a little cold water to work it into a dough. Chill the pastry for 30 min-
    utes before rolling it out to line a 26cm/10 inch flan tin or dish. Bake
    the pastry case blind for 10 minutes at 350°F/180°C/gas mark 4.
2   Meanwhile, steam or boil the broccoli florets until they have cooked
    through but are still a little crisp. Arrange them evenly over the bottom
    of the flan case, then sprinkle in the mushrooms and spread the garlic
    over the vegetables. Cover them with the cheese. Beat the eggs with
    the cream and season to taste with salt and freshly ground black

pepper. Pour this mixture into the flan case and bake it at 325°F/170°C/gas mark 3 for approximately 45 minutes or until the egg and cream mixture has set.

Prawn and Rice Ring

▶ **CHO 150g** ▶ **CALORIES 1440**   *serves 10*

Ring
175g/6oz/1 cup brown rice, cooked
275g/10oz/2½ cups frozen mixed vegetables, blanched

Dressing
4 x 15ml sp/4 tbs olive oil
2 x 15ml sp/2 tbs wine vinegar
pinch dry mustard
salt and freshly ground black pepper

Filling
2 x 15ml sp/2 tbs low-calorie mayonnaise
1 x 15ml sp/1 tbs tomato ketchup
few drops Worcestershire sauce
225g/8oz/2 cups prawns
lemon twist, to garnish

1   Add the vegetables to the rice. Then combine all the dressing ingredients in a screw-top jar and shake it well. Stir just enough of the dressing into the rice mixture to make it glisten, then spoon into a ring mould and press down into it well. Chill it well.

2   Meanwhile, make the filling. Combine the mayonnaise, ketchup, Worcestershire sauce and prawns and stir them all together well. Carefully turn the rice ring out onto a serving dish and fill the centre with the prawn mixture. Garnish it with a twist of lemon and serve.

Salmon Quiche

▶ CHO 910g ▶ CALORIES 1560   *serves 6*

Pastry

100g/4oz/1 cup wholemeal flour
50g/2oz/$\frac{1}{2}$ cup plain flour
pinch salt
50g/2oz/$\frac{1}{4}$ cup low-fat spread
25g/1oz/2 tbs white polyunsaturated fat
a little cold water to mix

Filling

1 x 200g/7oz can/1 cup pink salmon, drained and flaked
100g/4oz/$\frac{1}{2}$ cup cottage cheese, drained
2 size 3 eggs, lightly beaten
2 x 15ml sp/2 tbs skimmed milk
freshly ground black pepper
1 tomato, sliced

1   Make the pastry. Sieve the flours and salt into a bowl. Rub in the fats until the mixture resembles fine breadcrumbs. Stir in enough water to bind the mixture into a soft dough.

2   Chill the pastry for 30 minutes before rolling it out to line a 26cm/10 inch flan tin or dish. Bake the pastry case blind for 10 minutes at 400°F/200°C/gas mark 6. When it has cooked, spoon the flaked salmon evenly over the bottom.

3   Now make the filling. Liquidize or blend the cottage cheese, eggs, and milk until the mixture becomes smooth. Season it with freshly ground black pepper and pour it over the salmon. Arrange the tomato slices on top and bake at 400°F/200°C/gas mark 6 for 30–35 minutes or until the cheese, egg and milk mixture has set.

Mushroom and Onion Stuffing

▶ CHO 40g ▶ CALORIES 490

25g/1oz/2 tbs low-fat spread
1 x 15ml sp/1 tbs corn or sunflower oil
100g/4oz/1½ cups mushrooms, sliced
1 onion, peeled and chopped
100g/4oz/2 cups wholemeal breadcrumbs
1 x 15ml sp/1 tbs fresh parsley, chopped
salt and freshly ground black pepper
a little skimmed milk to bind, if necessary

1   Melt the low-fat spread and oil in a pan and lightly fry the mushrooms and onion until they have softened.
2   Transfer the mixture to a mixing bowl and stir in the remaining ingredients, seasoning with salt and freshly ground black pepper to taste. Make sure the ingredients are well combined. Stir in a little milk to bind the mixture if necessary.
3   Use to stuff a chicken or turkey.

Bread Sauce

▶ CHO 60g ▶ CALORIES 390   *makes approx 275ml/¹/₂ pint*

1 onion, peeled and quartered
425ml/³/₄ pint/2 cups skimmed milk
6 black peppercorns
1 bay leaf
1 blade mace
3 cloves
100g/4oz/2 cups fresh wholemeal breadcrumbs
pinch salt

1   Put the onion, milk, herbs and spices in a saucepan and bring to the boil.
2   Remove the pan from the heat, cover it tightly and leave it to infuse for 15–20 minutes.
3   Strain out the herbs and spices and return the milk to the pan once you have rinsed it out. Add the breadcrumbs and salt to taste.
4   Simmer the sauce gently to reheat the milk, stirring occasionally. Adjust the seasoning to taste just before serving.

Christmas Cake

▶ CHO 500g ▶ CALORIES 4360   *makes 36 portions*

175g/6oz/1 cup sultanas
175g/6oz/1 cup raisins
100g/4oz/^{2}/$_3$ cup currants
50g/2oz/^{1}/$_3$ cup glacé cherries, chopped
275ml/^{1}/$_2$ pint/1^1/$_3$ cups cold tea
200g/7oz/14 tbs polyunsaturated margarine
50g/2oz/^{1}/$_2$ cup ground almonds
275g/10oz/2^1/$_2$ cups wholemeal flour
2 x 5ml sp/2 tsp baking powder
2 x 5ml sp/2 tsp mixed spice
3 size 3 eggs, beaten
1 lemon, grated rind of
50g/2oz/^{1}/$_2$ cup blanched almonds, chopped

1   Put all the dried fruit into a bowl, cover it with the cold tea and leave
     the fruit to plump up overnight.
2   Cream the margarine and ground almonds until the mixture has light-
     ened in colour. Sieve the flour, baking powder and mixed spice into a
     bowl and then gradually add the eggs and half the flour mixture to the
     creamed mixture. Fold in the lemon rind and chopped nuts. Carefully
     fold the remaining flour into the fruit mixture to make a soft dropping
     consistency. Pour the mixture into a greased and lined 20cm/8 inch
     cake tin.
3   Bake the cake at 325°F/170°C/gas mark 3 for 1 hour then reduce the
     heat to 275°F/140°C/gas mark 1 for a further 1–1^1/$_4$ hours. Cover the
     top of the cake with greaseproof paper if it is browning too quickly.

4   To test whether the cake is done, push a clean skewer into the centre, leave it there for 2 seconds and if it comes out clean, the cake is cooked. Leave the cake to cool in its tin before turning it out. To store the cake, wrap it in foil or leave it 1 day to mature and then freeze it.

Marzipan

▶ CHO 80g ▶ CALORIES 950

100g/4oz/²/₃ cup ground almonds
50g/2oz/¹/₃ cup caster sugar
25g/1oz/¹/₄ cup white flour
1 size 3 egg

1   Beat all the ingredients together to form a smooth paste. You can do
     this by hand or use a food processor.
2   Divide the mixture into two and wrap it in cling film and store it in a
     cool place if you are not using it straight away.

▶ *Note to cooks* *This recipe makes enough marzipan to cover the top
and sides of an 18cm/7 inch cake.*

Dundee Cake

▶ CHO 340g ▶ CALORIES 2520   *makes 16 portions*

175g/6oz/³⁄₄ cup low-fat spread
50g/2oz/¹⁄₃ cup caster sugar
225g/8oz/2 cups fine wholemeal self-raising flour
pinch salt
1 x 5ml sp/1 tsp mixed spice
3 size 3 eggs, beaten
1 x 15ml sp/1 tbs skimmed milk
200g/7oz/1¹⁄₄ cups mixed fruit
25g/1oz/¹⁄₄ cup split almonds for decoration

1   Cream the low-fat spread and sugar until the mixture is light and fluffy. Mix the flour together with the salt and mixed spice. Add the eggs to the creamed mixture, one at a time, with a little of the flour mixture, stirring and then beating the mixture thoroughly after each addition. Stir in the milk and beat again. Add the fruit and the rest of the flour mixture, folding them in lightly.

2   Spoon the mixture into a greased and lined 18cm/7 inch round cake tin. Arrange the split almonds on top in the traditional pattern of concentric circles and bake for 1 hour at 350°F/180°C/gas mark 4 and for a further 1–1¹⁄₄ hours at 300°F/150°C/gas mark 2.

3   To check whether it is done, poke a clean skewer into the centre of the cake, leave it there for 2 seconds and, if when you remove it the skewer is clean, your cake is done. Then leave it to cool in the tin on a cooling rack before turning it out.

Mince Pies

▶ CHO 170g ▶ CALORIES 1150   *makes 12–16*

Pastry
100g/4oz/1 cup wholemeal flour
50g/2oz/½ cup plain flour
50g/2oz/¼ cup low-fat spread
25g/1oz/2 tbs white polyunsaturated vegetable fat
a little cold water to bind

Filling
4–4½ x 15ml sp/4–4½ tbs mincemeat
a little milk to glaze
a little powdered intense artificial sweetener

1   Make the pastry by sieving the flours together, rubbing in the fats until the mixture resembles breadcrumbs, then stir in a little water to make a soft dough.
2   Leave the pastry to chill in the refrigerator for 30 minutes, then roll it out on a lightly floured surface. Using a 5cm/2 inch pastry cutter and a small star cutter, cut out an equal number of bases and stars. Gather the scraps together and roll it out again to use the maximum amount of pastry.
3   Put the pastry circles in lightly greased patty tins and put 1 x 5ml sp/ 1 tsp of the mincemeat into each. Place a star on top of the mincemeat.
4   Bake the Mince Pies at 400°F/200°C/gas mark 6. When they are cooked, brush the stars with the milk and sprinkle a little of the sweetener over the top.

Christmas Pudding

▶ CHO 460g
▶ CALORIES 2920

makes 2 x 550ml/1 pint puddings;
each pudding serves 12

200g/7oz/4 cups wholemeal breadcrumbs
50g/2oz/$\frac{1}{3}$ cup dark brown sugar
100g/4oz/$\frac{1}{2}$ cup vegetable suet
pinch salt
1 x 5ml sp/1 tsp mixed spice
175g/6oz/1 cup sultanas
175g/6oz/1 cup raisins
100g/4oz/$\frac{2}{3}$ cup currants
25g/1oz/3 tbs blanched almonds, chopped
1 medium cooking apple, peeled, cored and grated
1 lemon, grated rind and juice of
1 size 3 egg, beaten
150ml/$\frac{1}{4}$ pint/$\frac{2}{3}$ cup Guinness
approx. 5 x 15ml sp/5 tbs skimmed milk, if necessary

1   Mix the dry ingredients with the lemon juice, egg and Guinness, mixing them together well. Add a little milk if the mixture is too stiff.
2   Pour the mixture into 2 550ml/1 pint pudding basins that have been lightly oiled. Cover them lightly with greaseproof paper and foil and steam for 2–3 hours or pressure cook at high pressure for 1–2 hours (consult the manufacturer's guide for your particular model).
3   Cover the puddings with fresh greaseproof paper and foil to store them. When you want to reheat them steam for 2 hours.

Stuffed Dates

▶ CHO 170g ▶ CALORIES 1050 *makes 16*

16 fresh dates
½ Marzipan recipe (see page 209)
16 petit four cases

1   Remove the stones from the dates, then fill each cavity with a little marzipan and put the date in a petit four case.

Easter Biscuits

▶ **CHO 190g** ▶ **CALORIES 1290**   *makes 28–30*

100g/4oz/¹⁄₃ cup low-fat spread
50g/2oz/¹⁄₃ cup sugar
1 size 3 egg, separated and white beaten
100g/4oz/1 cup wholemeal flour
50g/2oz/¹⁄₄ cup rice flour
1 x 5ml sp/1 tsp mixed spice
50g/2oz/¹⁄₃ cup currants
1 x 15ml sp/1 tbs skimmed milk, if necessary

1   Cream the low-fat spread and sugar together until the mixture is pale and creamy. Beat in the egg yolk then fold in the flours and mixed spice. Stir in the currants. If the dough is too stiff, mix in the milk to achieve a soft, pliable dough.

2   Knead the dough until it is smooth, then roll it out on a lightly floured surface. Cut out 28–30 rounds using a 5cm/2 inch pastry cutter. Gather the scraps together and roll it out again to waste as little dough as you can.

3   Place the biscuits on a lightly greased baking sheet and bake them in the centre of the oven at 400°F/ 200°C/gas mark 6 for about 10 minutes.

4   Brush the tops with the beaten egg white and return them to the oven to bake for about another 5 minutes. Cool them on a wire rack. When they have cooled, store them in an airtight container.

Hot Fruity Punch

▶ CHO 60g ▶ CALORIES 1890   *serves 12*

3 apples, cut into 8 pieces
3 oranges, cut into 8 pieces
12 whole cloves
2 cinnamon sticks
2 bottles red wine
550ml/1 pint/2½ cups dry sherry
550ml/1 pint/2½ cups unsweetened apple juice
1 orange, thinly sliced to decorate

1   Put the apple and orange pieces into a large pan with the cloves and
     cinnamon sticks and pour the red wine over them. Bring it to the boil
     and simmer, covered, for 10 minutes.
2   Remove the pan from the heat and let it stand for 10 minutes for the
     flavours to infuse.
3   Strain the wine and discard the spices, return the wine to the pan, pour
     in the apple juice and sherry and heat until the liquid starts to bubble
     at the edges of the pan.
4   Pour the wine into a warm serving bowl and float the orange slices on
     top. Serve immediately.

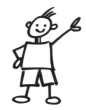

12 ideas for children

Children love to try different food, snacks, treats and drinks as much as adults do. As the majority of children are active and growing, it is even more important to provide them with healthy, nourishing meals. Quick food doesn't have to be junk food: why not try the American-style Hamburgers with the Bean Salad and homemade real Strawberry Milkshake?

You can make sure that there are plenty of protein foods in their diet by including meat, poultry, fish, dairy products, eggs and pulses. Vary what you give them and then you can be sure that they are eating a balanced diet and are less likely to become faddy eaters.

Sandwich Fillings

Skimmed Milk Cheese & Peanut Butter

▶ CHO 30g ▶ CALORIES 400

1 x 15ml sp/1 tbs crunchy peanut butter
2 x 15ml sp/2 tbs skimmed milk cheese or
2 tbs low-fat soft cheese
salt and freshly ground black pepper
2 slices wholemeal bread

1   Combine the ingredients, mixing them together well.
2   Spread the filling onto the bread.

Egg and Celery

▶ CHO 30g ▶ CALORIES 130

1 egg, hard-boiled
1 stick celery, finely chopped
1 x 15ml sp/1 tbs reduced-calorie mayonnaise
2 slices wholemeal bread

1   Mix the ingredients together, combining them well.
2   Spread the filling onto the bread.

Tuna and Mayonnaise
▶ CHO 30g ▶ CALORIES 200

100g/4oz/^{2}/$_3$ cup tinned tuna in brine, drained
2 x 15ml sp/2 tbs reduced-calorie mayonnaise
salt and freshly ground black pepper
a few slices cucumber and/or tomato
2 slices wholemeal bread

1   Combine the ingredients, mixing them well.
2   Spread the filling onto the bread.

Welsh Rarebit

▶ CHO 60g ▶ CALORIES 580   *serves 4*

4 slices wholemeal bread
100g/4oz/1 cup reduced-fat cheddar cheese, grated
pinch paprika
1 x 5ml sp/1 tsp mustard powder
1 x 5ml sp/1 tsp Worcestershire sauce

1   Toast the bread on one side under the grill.
2   Meanwhile, combine the remaining ingredients. Spread the cheese
    mixture on the untoasted side of the bread and grill gently for
    3–4 minutes until the cheese is bubbling and golden brown. Serve
    immediately.

American-style Hamburgers

▶ CHO 100g ▶ CALORIES 1270   *serves 4*

450g/1 lb extra lean mince beef
50g/2oz/1 cup wholemeal breadcrumbs
1 x 5ml sp/1 tsp mixed herbs
salt and freshly ground black pepper
1 size 3 egg, beaten
4 hamburger buns
4 lettuce leaves
2 tomatoes, sliced
1 onion, sliced

1   Put the minced beef, breadcrumbs and herbs into a bowl and mix
     them together well. Season to taste with salt and freshly ground black
     pepper, then bind the mixture together with the egg. Shape the
     mixture into 4 thick burgers and chill until needed.
2   Grill the burgers under medium heat for about 8 minutes on each side,
     or until they have cooked all the way through but aren't too dry. Then,
     split the buns and put a lettuce leaf and tomato and onion slices on
     the bottom half of each, put a burger on top then replace the other
     half of the bun.

Ham and Mushroom Stuffed Baked Potatoes

▶ CHO 30g ▶ CALORIES 650   *serves 4*

4 medium potatoes, cleaned
25g/1oz/2 tbs low-fat spread
1 onion, peeled and chopped
100g/4oz/1½ cups mushrooms, chopped
salt and freshly ground black pepper
50g/2oz/2 tbs lean ham, chopped
50g/2oz/½ cup reduced-fat cheddar cheese, grated

1   Bake the potatoes at 400°F/200°C/gas mark 6 for 45 minutes to 1
    hour, or until the potatoes are soft all the way through.
2   Towards the end of the potatoes' cooking time, melt the low-fat
    spread in a pan and sauté the onion and mushrooms. Season to taste
    and stir in the ham and grated cheese.
3   Cut the potatoes in half lengthways and scoop out the cooked flesh
    into a bowl, making sure that you do not pierce the skins. Mash it well,
    beat in the mushroom mixture, then spoon it back into the potato skins
    and return them to the oven and bake for a further 10–15 minutes.

Pizza

▶ CHO 150g ▶ CALORIES 1090   *serves 4–6*

Base
225g/8oz/2 cups wholemeal self-raising flour
1 x 5ml sp/1 tsp baking powder
pinch salt
25g/1oz/2 tbs low-fat spread
25g/1oz/¼ cup reduced-fat cheddar, grated
150ml/¼ pint/⅔ cup skimmed milk

Topping
2 x 15ml sp/2 tbs tomato purée
1 onion, peeled and finely chopped
pinch dried mixed herbs
50g/2oz/¾ cup button mushrooms, sliced
50g/2oz/½ cup reduced-fat cheddar, grated

1   Sieve the flour and baking powder into a bowl. Add the pinch of salt
    and the low-fat spread and rub them in until the mixture resembles
    coarse breadcrumbs. Stir in the cheese, then add the milk and mix
    until you have a rough dough.
2   Turn it out onto a floured surface and knead it until the dough is
    smooth. Roll it out on a lightly floured surface to form a 23cm/9 inch
    round, then transfer it to a lightly greased baking sheet.
3   Now add the topping. Spread the tomato purée over the surface,
    sprinkle on the onion and herbs, add the mushrooms, then sprinkle the
    cheese over the top.
4   Bake the pizza at 425°F/220°C/gas mark 7 for 20–25 minutes or until
    the cheese is bubbling and golden brown.

Strawberry and Yogurt Jelly

▶ CHO 10g ▶ CALORIES 90   *serves 4–6*

1 packet strawberry-flavour sugar-free jelly crystals
1 x 150g/5fl oz carton/²⁄₃ cup diet strawberry yogurt

1   Make up the jelly according to the directions on the packet and leave
    it to cool until it just starts to set, then fold in the yogurt. Pour
    the mixture into a wetted 550ml/1 pint mould or bowl, then chill in the
    refrigerator until it has set firm.
2   You can turn the jelly out onto a serving dish if you want to – just dip
    the mould in very hot water for a couple of seconds, invert the serving
    dish and put it on top of the mould, then, holding the plate tightly
    over it, turn it quickly and then lift the mould off.

Jelly Castles

▶ CHO 30g ▶ CALORIES 370 *serves 4*

1 packet orange-flavour sugar-free jelly crystals
4 x 15ml sp/4 tbs desiccated coconut
1 x 300g/10^{1}/$_{2}$oz can/1^{1}/$_{4}$ cups mandarin oranges in natural juice

1   Rinse out 4 150ml/^{1}/$_{4}$ pint moulds or empty yogurt cartons with cold water.
2   Make up the jelly according to the directions on the packet and pour equal amounts of the mixture into the wetted moulds. Cover them with clingfilm and chill until the jellies have set.
3   Unmould the jellies into individual dishes, dipping them briefly into very hot water.
4   Sprinkle the tops and sides of the jellies with the coconut and arrange all but 4 of the mandarin segments around the bottom edge of the jellies. Decorate the top of each jelly with a mandarin segment.
5   Chill the Jelly Castles until you are ready to serve.

▶ **Note to Cooks** *Use whichever flavour your child likes best and decorate with the appropriate fruit.*

Pear Mice

▶ CHO 40g ▶ CALORIES 180   *makes 6–7*

1 packet sugar-free jelly crystals
1 x 400g/14oz tin/1¾ cups pear halves in natural juice, drained and
   the juice reserved
18–21 currants
strip angelica

1   Make the jelly as per the instructions on the packet, using the pear
    juice made up to the amount given with water. Chill the jelly in the
    refrigerator until it has set.
2   Roughly chop the jelly and arrange it on a plate. Put the pear halves
    on the jelly, cut side down – these are the mice! Press the currants into
    the fruit so that each 'mouse' has 2 'eyes' and a 'nose'. Cut the angel-
    ica into very fine strips and stick a few into each side of the nose to
    make whiskers.

▶ **Note to Cooks** *This is ideal for children's parties and very easy to
make.*

Caribbean Drink

▶ CHO 50g ▶ CALORIES 220 *serves 4*

1 canned pineapple ring, in natural juice, drained
2 small bananas, peeled
1 wineglass unsweetened orange juice
1 lime, juice of
approx. 150ml/^{1}/$_4$ pint/^{2}/$_3$ cup diet pineapple and grapefruit drink
about 6 ice cubes

1   Put all the ingredients into a blender or liquidizer and process until the
     mixture is smooth.
2   Pour into 4 glasses and serve immediately.

Peach and Ginger Fizz

▶ CHO 30g ▶ CALORIES 130   *serves 4*

2 medium peaches, peeled, stoned and chopped
1 wineglass unsweetened apple juice
1 x 550ml/1 pint bottle/2½ cups slimline ginger ale
crushed ice

1   Put the peaches and apple juice in a blender or liquidizer and process until the mixture is smooth. Add the ginger ale.
2   Put the crushed ice into 4 glasses and pour out the drink. Serve immediately.

Strawberry Milkshake

▶ CHO 10g ▶ CALORIES 120   *serves 2*

275ml/½ pint/1⅓ cups skimmed milk
100g/4oz/1 cup strawberries, hulled if fresh, thawed if frozen
1 x 5ml sp/1 tsp intense artificial sweetener (optional)

1   Put the milk, strawberries and sweetener in a blender or liquidizer and
    process for 15–20 seconds.
2   Strain the milkshake into 2 glasses and serve immediately.

useful addresses

United Kingdom
British Diabetic Association, 10 Queen Anne Street, London W1M 0BD
020 7323 1531

The British Diabetic Association online
www.diabetes.org.uk

USA
American Diabetes Association, 1660 Duke Street, Alexandria, VA 22314
001-703 549 1500
1-800 232 3472 (USA Only)

Australia
Diabetes Australia, QBE Building, 33–35 Ainslie Avenue, Canberra ACT, PO
Box 944, Civic Square ACT 2608
61 62 475655
61 62 475722

Austria

Österreichischer Diabetikervereinigung, (Austrian Diabetes Association),
Moosstrasse 18, 5020 Salzburg
43 222 82 09 753

Belgium

Belgische Vereniging voor Suikerzieken, (Belgian Association for Diabetics),
BVS Secretariat, Charles de Kerchovelaan 369, B-9000 Ghent
32 91 20 05 20

Canada

Canadian Diabetes Association, 78 Bond Street, Toronto, Ontario M5B 2J8
1-416 362 4440

Czechoslovakia

Czechoslovak Diabetology Association, Internal Clinic ILF, National Diabetes
Program, Coordinating Centre, 762 75 Gottwaldov
42 28235

Denmark

Diabetesforeningen (Danish Diabetes Association), Filosofgangen 24,
5000 Odense C
45 66 129006

Finland

Suomen Diabetesliitto r.y. Diabetesförbundet i Finland r.f. (Finnish Diabetes
Association), Diabeteskeskus, Kirjoniementie 15, SF-33680 Tampere
358 31 600 333

France

Association Française des Diabétiques, 14 rue du Clos, 75020 Paris
331-40 08 24 25

Germany
Deutscher Diabetiker-Bund e.V. (German Diabetes Union), Danzigerweg 1,
D-5880 Lüdenscheid
49 2351 85053

Greece
Panhellenic Diabetic Association, Feidiou Street 18, Athens
30 1 362 9717

Hungary
Magyar Diabetes Társagág (Hungarian Diabetes Association), Korányi S. utca
2a, Budapest 1083
36 1 330 360

Ireland
Irish Diabetic Association, 82/83 Lower Gardiner Street, Dublin 1
363022

Italy
Associazione Italiana per la Difesa Degli, Interesi di Diabetici, Via del Scrofa
14, Roma
39 2 654 3784

Grand-Duché de Luxembourg
Association Luxembourgeoise du Diabète, PO Box 1316, Luxembourg
352 474545 / 352 4411 1

Netherlands
Diabetes Vereniging Nederland (Dutch Diabetes Association),
Puntenburgerlaan 91, 3812 CC, Amersfoort
31 33 63 05 66

Norway
Norges Diabetesforbund (Norwegian Diabetes Association), Østensjøveien
29, 0661 Oslo 6
47 2 65 45 50

Poland

Polskie Towarzystwo Diabetologiczne (Polish Diabetological Association), Kopernika 17, 31-501 Kraków
48 12 21 01 44
48 12 21 40 54

Portugal

Associaçao Protectora dos Diabéticos de Portugal (Portuguese Diabetic Association), Rua do Salitre, 118, 1200 Lisbon
351 1 680041 (42)
351 2 682729

Spain

Sociedad Espanola de Diabetes (Spanish Diabetes Society), Colegio Official de Médicos, Santa Isabel, 51, 28012 Madrid
341 2396519

Sweden

Svenska Endokrinolog föreningen (Swedish Society of Endocrinology), Department of Internal Medicine, University Hospital, S-75185 Uppsala
46 18 663000

Switzerland

(Switzerische Diabetes) Gesellschaft (Swiss Diabetes Association), Hegarstrasse 18, CH-8032 Zurich
41 1 383 13 15

Yugoslavia

Savez Drustava za Zastitu od Secerne Bolesti (The Association of Diabetic Societies of Yugoslavia), 4a Dugi Dol, PO Box 958, 41000 Zagreb
38 41 232 222
38 41 231 480

further reading

Day, Dr John, *The Diabetes Handbook, Insulin dependent diabetes* (1st Edition), Thorsons, 1986

Day, Dr John, *The Diabetes Handbook, Non-insulin dependent diabetes* (2nd Edition), British Diabetic Association, 1992

Govindji, Azmina and Jill Myers, *Diabetic Entertaining*, Thorsons, 1990

North, Judith, *Teenage Diabetes*, Thorsons, 1990

Sönksen, Peter, Charles Fox and Sue Judd, *Diabetes at your fingertips* (3rd Edition), Class Publishing, 1994

The British Diabetic Association

Diabetes affects just over two per cent of the UK population. Although it cannot be cured or prevented, it can be controlled by proper treatment. There may be times when you need advice or information and this is where the BDA can help.

The BDA is an independent registered charity with over 140,000 members and 400 local branches. It represents people with diabetes, liaising with Government Departments and professional bodies on matters concerning diabetes.

The Association provides information and practical advice for people with diabetes and their families. A wide range of literature, goods and videos are available on all aspects of diabetes.

The BDA's magazine, *Balance*, is published every two months and is sent free to members or is available from newsagents. It keeps readers up to date with the latest medical news, local events and includes articles on living with diabetes. All people with diabetes are advised to eat healthily and *Balance* gives recipes and dietary information to help bring interest and variety to diabetic eating.

The Association also supports research to improve treatments and to find a prevention or cure for diabetes. Currently spending around £3.5 million each year, the BDA is the largest single contributor dedicated to diabetic research.

For over 60 years, the BDA has strived to achieve its aims, but it has only been able to do so with the help of its members and supporters. Please join the BDA. For further details and an application form, contact:

British Diabetic Association
10 Queen Anne Street
London W1M 0BD
United Kingdom
Tel: 020 7323 1531
www.diabetes.org.uk

index

adaptations 33–4
addresses 229–32, 235
alcohol 17, 18–19, 28, 29
American Diabetes Association 20, 229
American-style Hamburgers 216, 220
apples
    Apple Delight 170
    Baked Apples 161
    Eve's Pudding 160
apricots 172
artificial sweeteners 12–13, 21
aubergines 150–1
Autumn Salad 132
avocados 48

baked dishes
    Apples 161
    Fish 74
    Fish with Pepper Sauce 87
Bakewell Tart 162–3

baking 33–6, 181–99
Balance magazine 234
Banana and Walnut Slices 35, 186
Barbecued Pork Chops 71
beans 6–7, 32, 35, 50
    Bean Salad 216
    Bean and Vegetable Stew 104
    Chickpea Moussaka 105–6
    Italian Bean Salad 130
    Mixed Bean Hot Pot 107
    Mung Bean and Vegetable Cottage Pie 111
    Red Kidney Beans with Walnuts 131
    Three-Bean Cassoulet 103
bedtimes 22, 24, 28
beef
    American-style Hamburgers 220
    Beef Stew and Dumplings 68–9
    Beefburger Surprise 61
    Carbonade of Beef 70

Cottage Pie 62
Macaroni Mince 63
Minced Beef Cobbler 60
Moussaka 65–6
Spaghetti Bolognese 64
blood sugar 5–7, 11, 19, 27–30
blurred vision 3
boiled potatoes 5, 7, 35–6
braised dishes
Celery 145
Green Lentils 108
bread
Bread Sauce 206
Date and Walnut Loaf 190
Tea Bread 187
Wholemeal Bread 182
breakfasts 22, 23
British Diabetic Association (BDA) 1,
8, 20, 229, 234–5
broccoli
Broccoli in Ham and Cheese Sauce
53
Broccoli and Mushroom Flan
201–2
Butter Icing 199
Butterfly Cakes 185

cabbage 146
calories 9–17, 19, 26
adaptations 34
calculations 33
desserts 159
Canadian Diabetes Association 20,
230
carbohydrates 13, 19–21, 28
calculations 32–3

emergencies 29
Carbonade of Beef 70
Caribbean Drink 226
Celebration Cake 189
celery 145
cheese
Cheese and Fruit Cocktail 156
Cheese Sauce 126
Cheesy Leek and Potato Casserole
116
Cheesecake 174
chicken
Chicken Breasts with Pineapple
Sauce 58
Chicken Broth 44
Chicken Liver Pâté 46
Lemon and Herb Baked Chicken
57
Stir-fried Chicken with Cashews 56
Sweet and Sour Chicken 55
Chickpea Moussaka 6, 105–6
chicory 144
children 216–28
CHO allowances 34
CHO exchange 20–1
cholesterol 6, 8–9, 19
Christmas 200
Christmas Cake 207–8
Christmas Pudding 212
Cinnamon Scone 196
constipation 6
Cooked Chicory 144
Cottage Pie 62
courgettes
Courgette and Sweetcorn Gratin
10, 112–13

Courgettes á la Grecque 153
Curd Cheese Topping 198

dairy products 10, 35, 216
Date and Walnut Loaf 190
desserts 2, 11, 27, 35, 159–80
diabetes
    associations 4–5, 229–32
    introduction 3–30
    products 21
Diabetes Australia 20, 229
dieticians 14, 17, 20, 29
dips 37
dressings 9, 140–1, 152
drinks 11, 12, 21, 216, 226–8
Dundee Cake 210

Easter Biscuits 214
eating out 25–8
eggs 9, 216
    Pancakes 124–6
    Welsh Rarebit 219
elderly people 1
emergencies 29, 30
Europe 20, 229–32
Eve's Pudding 160
exchange lists 20
eye problems 4

Fairy Cakes 184
fast food joints 25, 26
fats 6, 8–11, 13
    adaptations 33–5
    ingredients 31
feelings 4–5
festive occasions 200–15

fibre 5–7, 11, 17, 37
    desserts 159
    ingredients 31
    meat 50
fillings
    pancakes 125–6
    sandwiches 217–18
fish 10, 35, 72–95
    children 216
    Fish Cakes 95
    Fish Creole 90
    fish oils 9
    Fish Salad Platter 137
    Fish Steaks and Peppercorn Sauce
        91
    Fish-Stuffed Baked Potatoes 78
flour 33, 36
foot problems 4
Fresh Fruit Jelly 175
fried foods 6, 8, 10, 35
fruit 7, 8
    Fresh Fruit Jelly 175
    Fruit Fool 177
    Fruit and Vegetable Mixed Salad
        138
    Fruit and Yogurt Whips 168

genital itching 3
glucose 3
gooseberries 167
Grape Jelly 178
Greek-style Lamb Kebabs 59
Guacamole 48

haddock
    Haddock Crumble 82

Haddock and Vegetable Casserole 86
Kedgeree 80
Smoked Haddock Plait 75
Ham and Cheese Sauce 53
healthy eating 1, 5–25
holidays 25, 27–8
Hot Fruity Punch 215
hypoglycaemia 6, 29

ice cream 176
icing 199
identification 29
illness 30
ingredients 31–2
injections 3, 4, 17, 28–9
insulin 3–4, 6, 17, 20, 27–30
Italian Bean Salad 130

Jam Tarts 195
Jelly Castles 224

Kedgeree 80
kidney problems 4

lamb
    Greek-style Lamb Kebabs 59
    Navarin of Lamb 67
Leeks in Curry Dressing 152
Lemon and Herb Baked Chicken 57
lentils 6–7, 32, 35
    Braised Green Lentils 108
    Lentil Moussaka 109–10
    Lentil Soup 42
lettuce 157
liver 3

Low-Calorie French Dressing 140
low-fat foods 10, 35
lunches 22, 23, 127

Macaroni Mince 63
mackerel
    Mackerel with Lime 79
    Mackerel with Mustard and Oats 89
    Mediterranean-style Mackerel 49
    Smoked Mackerel Pâté 45
Madeleines 194
Maids of Honour 193
Marbled Apricots 172
Marzipan 209
mashed potatoes 5, 7
meat 10, 35, 50–71, 216
medication 6, 13
Mediterranean-style Mackerel 49
Mince Pies 211
Minced Beef Cobbler 60
Minestrone Soup 39–40
Mixed Bean Hot Pot 7, 107
Mixed Vegetable Curry 117–18
monounsaturated fats 8–10, 35
motivation 14, 15, 16
Moussaka 65–6
Mung Bean and Vegetable Cottage Pie 111
mushrooms
    Mushroom and Onion Stuffing 205
    Mushrooms á la Grecque 154
    Stuffed Mushrooms 147
Mustard Dressing 141

Navarin of Lamb 67

nerve problems 4
Nut Roast 123

oats 6
oily fish 72
okra 149
olive oil 9, 10, 35
overweight people 4, 8, 11, 13,
    15–18

packaged foods 11
Pancakes 124–6
pancreas 3
Paprika Fish 77
parents 1
pasta
    Pasta and Pesto Sauce 97
    Red Lentil Lasagne 100–1
    Vegetable Lasagne 98–9
    Wholewheat Pasta Salad 128
pâtés 37
peaches
    Peach and Ginger Fizz 227
    Peach Ice Cream 176
    Peach Pudding 164
pears
    Pear Mice 225
    Pears Cassis 173
    Pears in Mulled Wine 179
    Stuffed Pears 47
peas 7, 35
peppers
    Peppers á la Provence 148
    Stuffed Pepper 122
    Stuffed Peppers and Tomatoes
        51–2

Pineapple Sauce 58
Pizza 222
plaice 85
Plate Model 24–5
polyunsaturated fats 8–10, 35
pork 71
    Pork Stir-fry 54
potatoes 5, 7–8, 32, 35
    Cheesy Leek and Potato Casserole
        116
    Fish-Stuffed Baked Potatoes 78
    Ham and Mushroom Stuffed
        Baked Potatoes 221
    Potato and Sprout Bake 143
poultry 10, 35, 50–71, 216
prawns
    Prawn and Cashew Nut Curry 76
    Prawn and Rice Ring 203
    Prawn and Rice Salad 136
    Rice with Prawns 88
processed foods 10
protein 7, 9, 11, 13, 216
Prune and Nut Cake 191
puddings 2, 35, 159–80

raspberries
    Raspberry and Kiwi Whip 35, 166
    Raspberry Mousse 171
reading list 233
recipes
    calculations 32–3
    introduction 31–6
Red Kidney Beans with Walnuts 131
Red Lentil Lasagne 10, 100–1
refined foods 7
restaurants 25, 27

Summer Pudding 180
suppers 22, 24
support 14
Sweet and Sour Chicken 55
Sweetcorn and Mushroom Filling 126

talking 5
Taramasalata 38
Tea Bread 187
thirst 3
Three-Bean Cassoulet 103
tips 35–6
tiredness 3
tomatoes
    Stuffed Peppers and Tomatoes
        51–2
    Tomato Soup 41
tooth decay 11, 12
Trifle 165
trout 84
Tsatziki 142
Tuna Sauce 73
Turkey Broth 44
Type 1 diabetes 3
Type 2 diabetes 3–4

urine 3, 30

vegans 1

vegetables 8, 37
    Mixed Vegetable Curry 117–18
    Savoury Crumble 120–1
    Stir-Fried Vegetable Salad 119
    Summer Vegetable Salad 155
    Vegetable Casserole 115
    Vegetable Lasagne 98–9
    Vegetable Rice 158
vegetarian dishes 1, 96–126
Vegetarian Paella 102
Victoria Sandwich 35, 183

Waldorf Salad 129
water 7
Watercress and Onion Soup 43
weight
    chart 16–18
    watching 1–3, 6, 13, 15
weights and measures 32
Welsh Rarebit 219
white fish 72
Wholemeal Bread 182
Wholewheat Pasta Salad 128
World Health Organisation (WHO) 8

yogurt
    Yogurt Gooseberry Fool 35, 167
    Yogurt Snow with Raspberry Sauce
        169

Rhubarb and Raisin Cake 188
rice 36
    Prawn and Rice Ring 203
    Prawn and Rice Salad 136
    Rice and Millet Salad 134–5
    Rice Salad 133
    Vegetable Rice 158
    Vegetarian Paella 102
Rich Scones 197
Rock Cakes 192

Sailor's Pie 81
salads 127–58
salmon
    Salmon Parcels 94
    Salmon Quiche 204
salt 6, 17–18, 35
Sandwich Fillings 217–18
saturated fats 8–9, 33
sauces
    Bread 206
    Cheese 126
    Ham and Cheese 53
    Pepper 87
    Peppercorn 91
    Pesto 97
    Pineapple 58
    Raspberry 169
    Tuna 73
    Yogurt 84
Sautéed Okra 149
Savoury Crumble 120–1
shopping 15
side dishes 127–58
Slimmer's Salad 139
slimming 14–15

Smoked Haddock Plait 75
Smoked Mackerel Pâté 9, 45
snacks 10, 22, 24, 27–9, 127, 216
soluble fibre 6, 19
soups 37–49
Spaghetti Bolognese 64
specialist products 21
Spring Cabbage 146
starch 3, 5–6, 11, 17, 19
starters 37–49
Steamed Fish and Vegetables 9
Steamed Trout with Yogurt Sauc
stir-fries 26
    Chicken with Cashews 56
    Pork 54
    Vegetable Salad 119
    Vegetables 114
strawberries
    Strawberry Milkshake 216, 2
    Strawberry and Yogurt Jelly
students 1
stuffed dishes
    Aubergines 150–1
    Dates 213
    Iceberg Lettuce 157
    Mushrooms 147
    Pears 47
    Pepper 122
    Peppers and Tomatoes 51–
    Plaice 85
stuffing 205
sugar 6, 11–13, 17, 21
    adaptations 34
    desserts 159
    ingredients 32
Summer Fish 92

Rhubarb and Raisin Cake 188
rice 36
    Prawn and Rice Ring 203
    Prawn and Rice Salad 136
    Rice and Millet Salad 134–5
    Rice Salad 133
    Vegetable Rice 158
    Vegetarian Paella 102
Rich Scones 197
Rock Cakes 192

Sailor's Pie 81
salads 127–58
salmon
    Salmon Parcels 94
    Salmon Quiche 204
salt 6, 17–18, 35
Sandwich Fillings 217–18
saturated fats 8–9, 33
sauces
    Bread 206
    Cheese 126
    Ham and Cheese 53
    Pepper 87
    Peppercorn 91
    Pesto 97
    Pineapple 58
    Raspberry 169
    Tuna 73
    Yogurt 84
Sautéed Okra 149
Savoury Crumble 120–1
shopping 15
side dishes 127–58
Slimmer's Salad 139
slimming 14–15

Smoked Haddock Plait 75
Smoked Mackerel Pâté 9, 45
snacks 10, 22, 24, 27–9, 127, 216
soluble fibre 6, 19
soups 37–49
Spaghetti Bolognese 64
specialist products 21
Spring Cabbage 146
starch 3, 5–6, 11, 17, 19
starters 37–49
Steamed Fish and Vegetables 93
Steamed Trout with Yogurt Sauce 84
stir-fries 26
    Chicken with Cashews 56
    Pork 54
    Vegetable Salad 119
    Vegetables 114
strawberries
    Strawberry Milkshake 216, 228
    Strawberry and Yogurt Jelly 223
students 1
stuffed dishes
    Aubergines 150–1
    Dates 213
    Iceberg Lettuce 157
    Mushrooms 147
    Pears 47
    Pepper 122
    Peppers and Tomatoes 51–2
    Plaice 85
stuffing 205
sugar 6, 11–13, 17, 21
    adaptations 34
    desserts 159
    ingredients 32
Summer Fish 92

Summer Pudding 180
suppers 22, 24
support 14
Sweet and Sour Chicken 55
Sweetcorn and Mushroom Filling 126

talking 5
Taramasalata 38
Tea Bread 187
thirst 3
Three-Bean Cassoulet 103
tips 35–6
tiredness 3
tomatoes
    Stuffed Peppers and Tomatoes
        51–2
    Tomato Soup 41
tooth decay 11, 12
Trifle 165
trout 84
Tsatziki 142
Tuna Sauce 73
Turkey Broth 44
Type 1 diabetes 3
Type 2 diabetes 3–4

urine 3, 30

vegans 1

vegetables 8, 37
    Mixed Vegetable Curry 117–18
    Savoury Crumble 120–1
    Stir-Fried Vegetable Salad 119
    Summer Vegetable Salad 155
    Vegetable Casserole 115
    Vegetable Lasagne 98–9
    Vegetable Rice 158
vegetarian dishes 1, 96–126
Vegetarian Paella 102
Victoria Sandwich 35, 183

Waldorf Salad 129
water 7
Watercress and Onion Soup 43
weight
    chart 16–18
    watching 1–3, 6, 13, 15
weights and measures 32
Welsh Rarebit 219
white fish 72
Wholemeal Bread 182
Wholewheat Pasta Salad 128
World Health Organisation (WHO) 8

yogurt
    Yogurt Gooseberry Fool 35, 167
    Yogurt Snow with Raspberry Sauce
        169